GW00724823

Aspire

Aspire works with people with spinal
cord injuries to create opportunity,
choice and independence.

INTRODUCTION

Spinal injury doesn't discriminate - it can happen to anyone at any time. So the people you will meet in this book have not been picked in any sort of attempt to reflect perfectly the spinally injured population; instead there are men and women, young and old, some who have gone on to achieve outstanding sporting excellence and others who have never been near a basketball court in their lives. Much like, in fact, any random sample of 25 people from any high street in the country.

As a national charity, Aspire's Services are there for everyone who has a spinal cord injury. We're delighted that this book will add to our existing projects and be available to patients and their families throughout the UK and Ireland, not least because its very concept stems from conversations Aspire staff have had with many people who have been affected by spinal cord injury. All of them have been looking for the chance to hear from individuals who have sat where they are sitting, who know what it feels like and can give the reassurance that can sometimes be so hard to find.

Over the 26 years since we were founded, Aspire has helped literally thousands of people regain their independence. In doing so, we have learned, above all, that we work with individuals. This book is a celebration of that individuality.

As I talked to the 25 people featured here the differences between them constantly surprised me. Some chose to spare me the nitty-gritty, others felt I should get the full gory details; some were self confessed grumps while others never stopped telling jokes and laughing. One thing they all had in common was that they all wanted to share their story; to say, "It's my life and this is how I'm living it."

Few of us know what we would do if we, or a loved one, had a spinal cord injury. You are probably reading this because you do know. I can only say that if glancing through these stories by those who have been there before gives you hope, maybe inspiration or just makes you smile then our efforts have been worthwhile.

Angi Jones
Vice President

2

PREFACE

During my nine years' involvement with Aspire, I have learnt two things above all others about this charity; that its essential 'can-do' message to people who sustain spinal cord

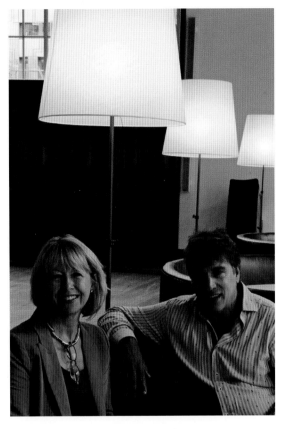

injuries is a positive and empowering one, and that it works.

Hosting Aspire's Sports Quiz Dinner, an annual fund-raising event the charity organises at Lord's Cricket Ground in London, I have had the opportunity to meet and listen to many remarkable individuals who, following a spinal cord injury and with Aspire's help, have gone on to achieve remarkable things - sailing single-handed round Britain, breaking world land speed records, winning Paralympic medals. But just as clear in my memory are the faces and stories of those individuals whose achievements following injury have been less headline-grabbing but just as significant – men and women who have achieved the goal they set themselves, whether it be to go back to the job they have always loved, or to support their families practically, emotionally and financially, or to change careers and find something that really satisfies them, or to marry and have children. In short, they've achieved all the aspirations that we all have and which, they tell me, seem suddenly out of reach in that moment when you wake up to find yourself in a spinal injury centre.

This book of personal stories brings all those conversations back to me. What follows is both an inspiration and a testament to the determination of the individuals concerned.

John Inverdale
Patron

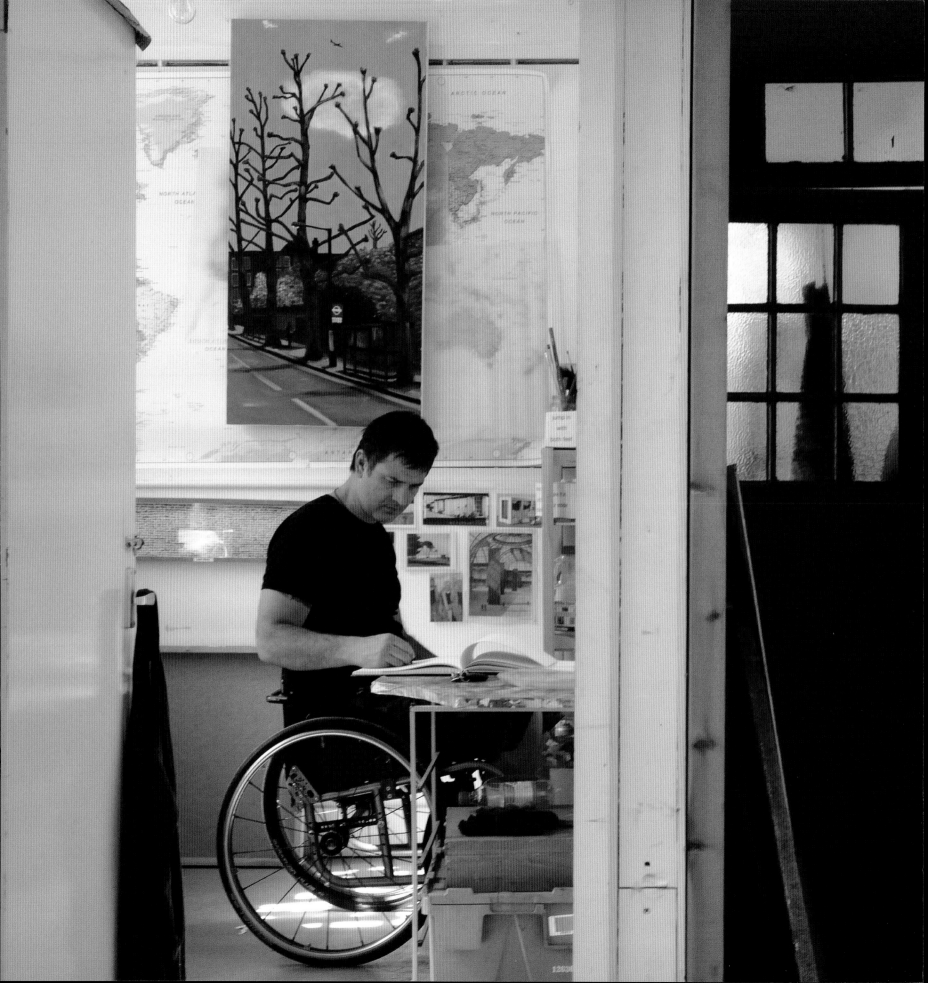

My wife was pregnant at the time of my accident and I was determined to be by her side for the birth. I was one of the earliest releases ever from the spinal unit and I was able to wheel myself into the birthing room and welcome our daughter, Rosalie, into the world. The safe delivery was wonderful but we had a problem to overcome: where to live while our flat was adapted? That is where Aspire's Housing Scheme came in. The Aspire house we lived in was in Edgware, North London, and had originally been converted for the charity by Anneka Rice as part of one of her television programmes.

Of course I'm interested in research into 'the cure', but realise it's unlikely I'll benefit from any results as my lesion is 95 per cent complete. From what I understand, any possible cures in the foreseeable future will be more likely to benefit those with incomplete injuries. Another important area of research is around the psychology of how to make the best of your situation and also, as the years go by, around the ageing issues wheelchair users will have to face. If you focus on what may happen, you can lose focus on living in the 'now'.

I wrote a book, *Looking up*, and also wrote a regular column for the Times newspaper, both of which helped me to come to terms with my injury. I had been a highly active, six foot tall, outdoors character and wanted to convey an accurate account of the overwhelming feelings of anger and despair, of how I have rebuilt my life and how my work as an artist is developing and another chapter in my life is opening.

Find a way to do it and then decide if it's worth doing

I've used callipers but I'm tall and if I fall I could do more damage and perhaps be unable to push my wheelchair. You only have to visit the seaside and try pushing a chair on sand to realise how incredibly efficient human beings are walking the way they do.

I do miss the physical life I enjoyed before my injury, but I still play sport frequently, especially tennis. And I still get into the great outdoors with my family whenever possible.

I guess my attitude is best summed up as: "Find a way to do it and then decide if it's worth doing."

I'm a very competitive person. So when a physio told me I'd never be able to back wheel balance, I stayed awake all night practising until I could do it. Now I teach wheelchair skills, and that's where I met my boyfriend. He is also in a wheelchair, which is really supportive in lots of ways. We have a great time together and travel a lot; we've been to Africa twice now. It's the small things that are important though, like always being at the same level as each other.

I had my accident when I was out sailing in the Atlantic with my best friend. I had just completed a sketch of a lighthouse when I was thrown across the boat. At first I was in hospital in Portugal while they put lots of bolts, plates and bone grafts into my neck. I was brought home by Lear Jet (how cool!) and everything seemed fine.

Then I found myself in the high-dependency unit. It was a really dark room and it seemed that they just left me there. And so it hit me, what had happened to me and how serious it was. I felt so alone in my body, distraught and in absolute misery.

Soon after leaving hospital I did an art foundation course at a totally inaccessible college, though really I was still thinking about what I was going to do in life. I still am! My accident was only a few years ago so it's still early days. In some ways I'm really sorted, but I realise now that it's a state of mind that I come in and out of. I would like to find a career but there's still plenty of other stuff I want to do first, like travel. I want to do more drawing and painting too, but now I need to be in the right place with an accessible studio.

Then I turned to drink

When I was in hospital I totally lost my appetite, and it's still something that I have problems with. But, perhaps as a result of having to pay attention to what I eat, I've now become a real 'foodie'. I love cooking and am always trying new recipes. I've also turned to drink by enrolling on a wine tasting course which is brilliant. It's creative and I'm not restricted by my injury. Whilst waiting to do the diploma I'm planning a road trip to the Champagne region, and then we'll see how accessible those châteaux are!

My life has changed, but then it was always going to. I don't look back; I wouldn't if I weren't in a wheelchair. I see my life in two separate blocks, before and after, and it's me who joins them both.

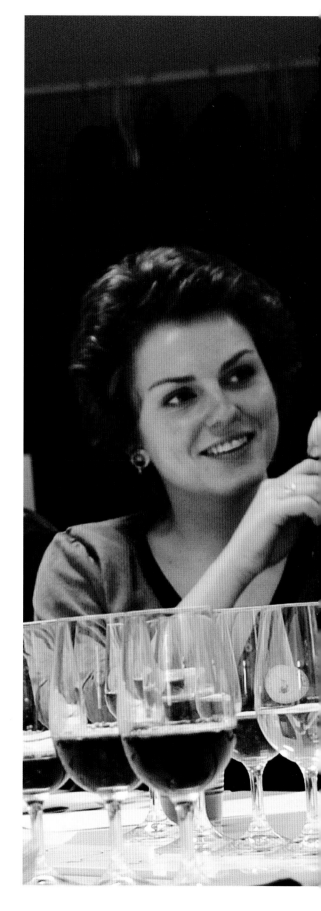

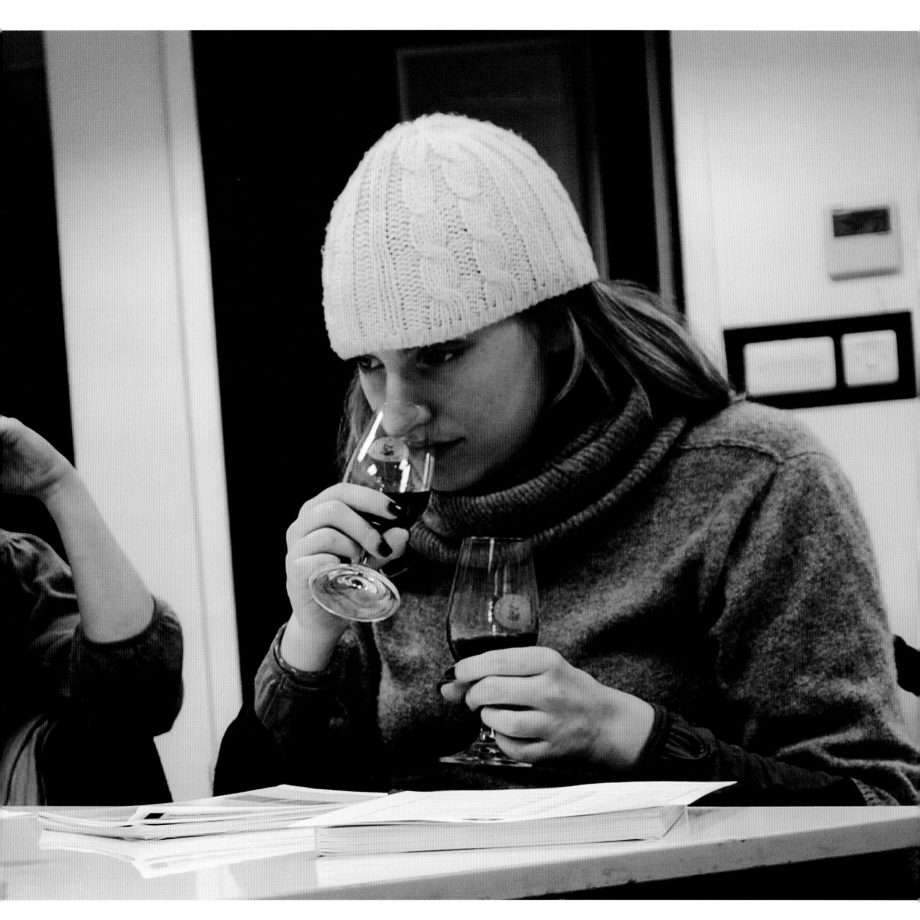

My friends and family used to describe me as a Billy the Whizz-type character. I ran businesses, played a myriad of sports, travelled the world and seemed never to be in the same place for more than five minutes.

In January of 2006 I was on the holiday of a lifetime, celebrating the New Year in Goa. My friends and I were on a sunset walk on the beach when I fancied a swim; I plunged into the sea and hit a sandbank. I was conscious for the initial couple of minutes and knew immediately that I had broken my neck. As the water around me turned red with the blood pouring from my head, I began to mentally say goodbye to all the people that I loved; my family, girlfriend, friends and my five beautiful godchildren.

Hospitals in India aren't exactly BUPA standard! I could order a beer but beyond that I didn't speak the language and being there brought its own set of challenges. It was deliriously hot and each time I regained consciousness I found myself either next to a bed hosting a recently deceased body, or looking at a sacred cow which had wandered into the intensive care unit. The doctors gave me a one per cent chance of survival.

The love and support from friends and family is what gets you through; we've all cried and laughed at the extremities this injury imposes on me. And they treat me exactly the same as before; the guys even used to come into the hospital wearing my best clothes, claiming I wouldn't be needing them for a while after all the weight I'd lost in India! This may seem callous but it was all about sustaining the same banter we've always had.

I went home to the same non-adapted property that I had lived in before the accident. It's needed lots of work, including ramps, changes to the driveway, widening doors, new flooring, ceiling track hoists and so on. Two years on and it's nearly there.

I love my life so it's good to have proved the doctors wrong. Life is getting back to normal and once again I find myself very busy, completing a counselling course, travelling, working and just about fitting in the time to go skiing. I hope and believe I'm still the same Billy the Whizz character I've always been.

The guys treat me exactly the same as they did before

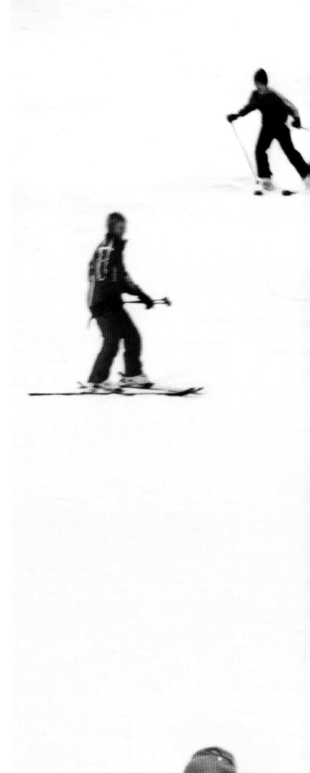

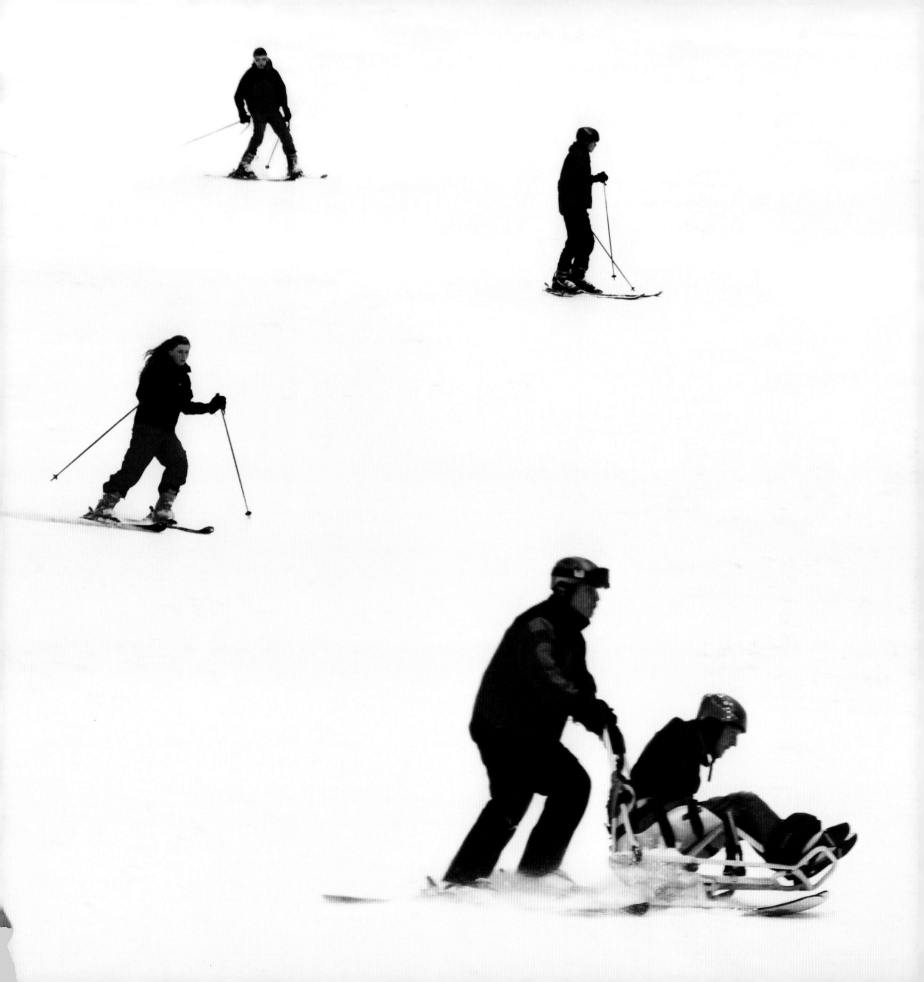

I had just moved to London when I had my accident. My back was broken when a drunk plunged 40 feet on top of me as I left my firm's 1986 office Christmas party. Of course, my parents wanted me to move back in with them, but I was determined not to live in a granny flat in Stafford. So, when some friends offered me a room in their flat, I jumped at the chance. It turned out to be a great decision as I really had to learn to do things for myself.

Working for Aspire helped me with my confidence and made me feel better about myself. I am now happily married to Chris and we have two lovely children. Although I had known Chris for a long time, we did not get married until I was 33. The doctors had told me straight after my injury that I could still have children but I wasn't sure I wanted them then. Of course, once I was married, I did, and Emily came first. I then miscarried but, after fertility treatment, I had Ollie when I was 38 (quite old, evidently, to be a mother when you are a wheelchair user).

I thought the doctors would want to do caesareans for both babies, but they said I could have a natural childbirth as my injury is quite low and I would find it too difficult to manoeuvre my wheelchair after the surgery. I have a steel rod in my spine, so they couldn't give me an epidural, and both children were induced - with the aid of some gas and air. Of course I had worries about being a mum and I wasn't looking forward to having to let other people do the things for my children that I couldn't. But the worry was worse than the reality and I just had to find new ways to do things, like finding a cot which came down low enough for me to lift my baby.

I love travelling and Chris and I are taking the children to Lapland to see Father Christmas. I'm always setting new goals for myself: I've tried skiing (I'm building up to a challenging black run), bungee jumping, parachute jumping, hydro speeding, para gliding and karate. I also love hot, sunny holidays but beaches are a challenge to any wheelchair user. Even when there are challenges, though, my friends have helped me not to be selfish and to be more considerate of others. Together with my husband and family, they've got me through. I just keep as active as I can - I can't be doing with unhappy.

I can't be doing with unhappy

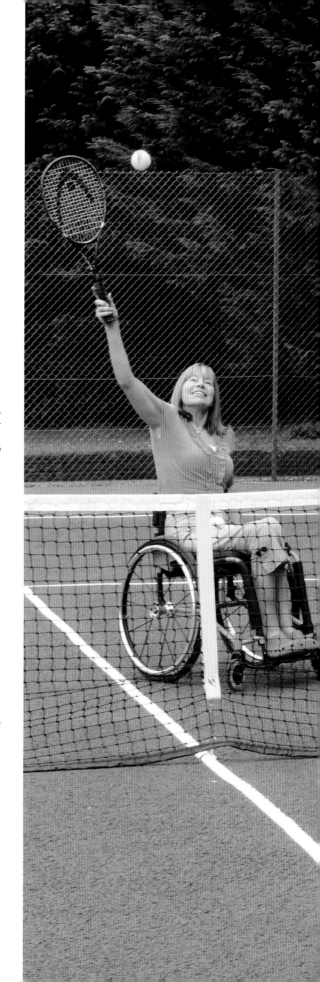

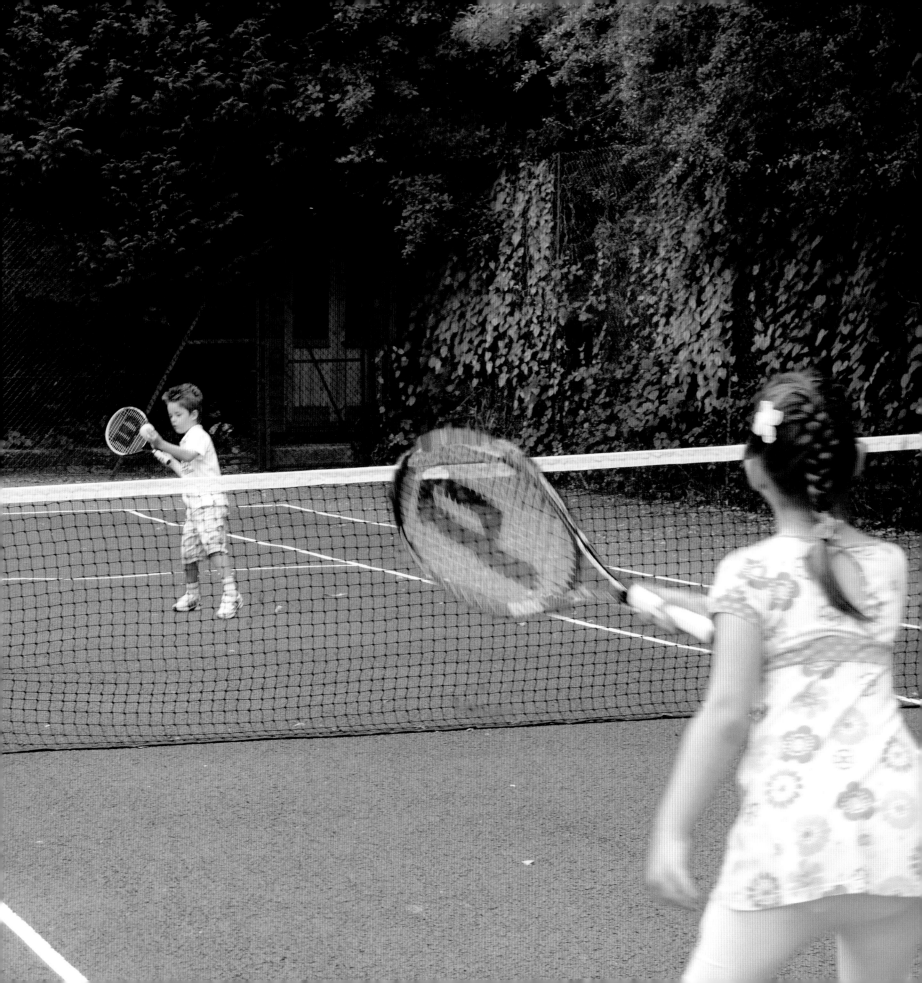

I was in my mid 60s when I had a fall and broke my leg. I found crutches really difficult to cope with, so I hobbled about and probably twisted my spine because, a few weeks later as I turned to dry my hands, an awful pain shot down my leg. A disk had imploded and I was unable to move my legs, which is why I am in a wheelchair. In some ways I consider myself very fortunate; if this had happened when I was younger I think it would have been much more difficult for me to cope with.

I used to do lots of gardening but now I have some pots on the terrace and I just keep an eye on the rest of the garden. We thought of raising the flower beds, but it seemed such an upheaval just for me. I lose myself in reading, it's such a great escape, and I've learnt how to use a computer with Aspire in one of their assistive technology suites. I find the internet marvellous; I spend time online on Google or shopping for all sorts of things. I have also researched our family ancestry and got quite a long way with it, but I have now handed it on to the children to continue; it was taking up so much time!

My weekly swim in the excellent Aspire pool at Stanmore has been my lifeline. My husband drives me to the Centre, then I take myself off to change and do my lengths while he goes to the gym and exercises. We meet up again for lunch in the café afterwards – both fairly shattered but knowing it's done some good.

> I try to keep happy and optimistic, but sometimes I get frustrated

I try to keep happy and optimistic. I do sometimes get very frustrated and cross with myself but try to be grateful when people help me, even when it's something I could do on my own. I remember years ago visiting some elderly people in a home and realising how difficult it was to spend time with someone who was miserable and complaining, whereas everyone enjoyed being with people who smiled and had a cheerful outlook. I think it is vital to accept what has happened to you and look forward, realising you are not the only person in the world that this has happened to.

As my Mother used to quote: "Laugh and the whole world laughs with you; weep, and you weep alone."

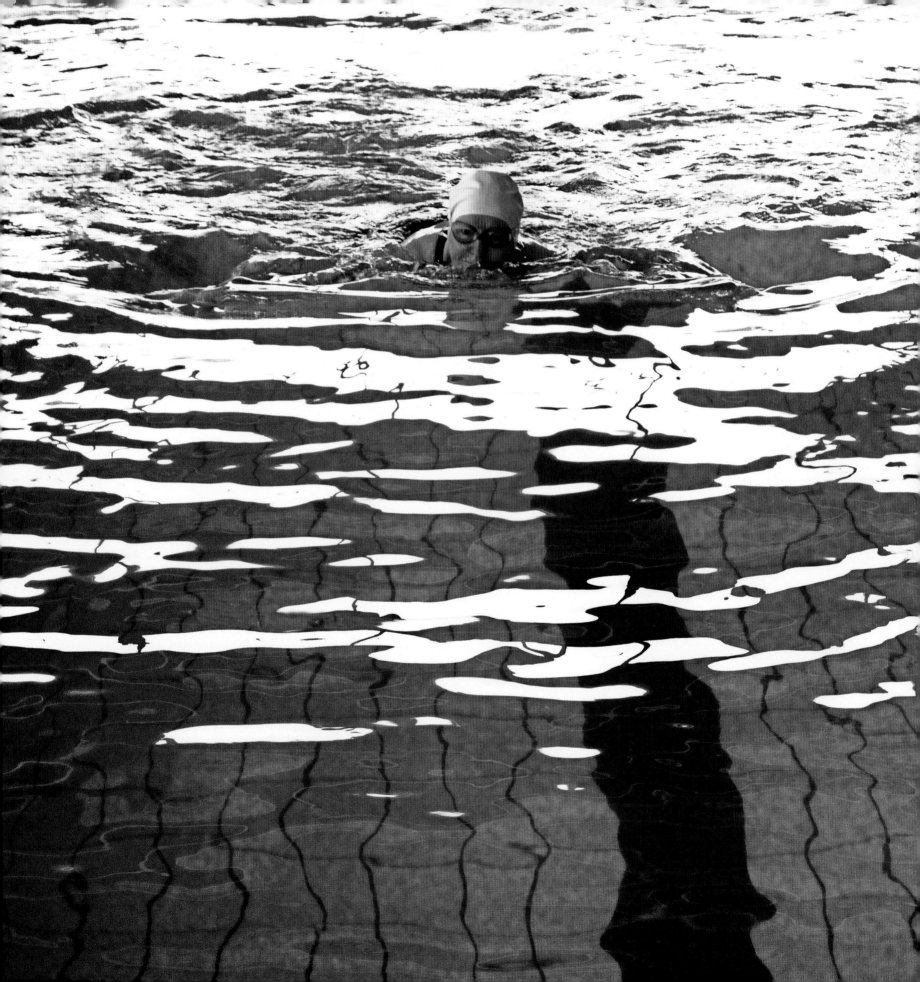

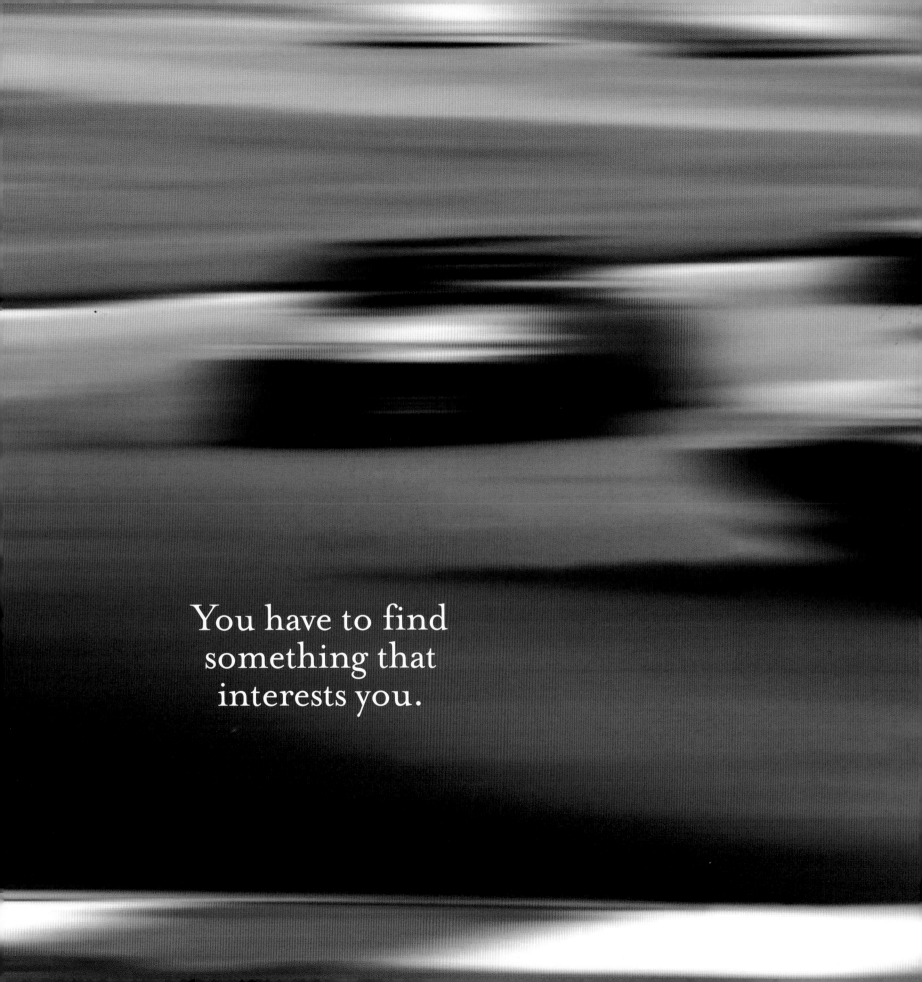

You have to find
something that
interests you.

At the time of my injury, my daughter was only three months old and I was the Managing Director and shareholder in an international insurance brokerage. I was determined to get back to my family and work as soon as possible so worked really hard at my physio and rehab. I was released from the Spinal Centre after just three months.

Despite my strong determination to get on with what was a successful career, life was to change further. My employer wanted to renegotiate my contract and cut my pay in half. I wasn't going to agree to that, so I left and joined another broker. Today I own the whole company.

I might not be the most mobile person, but I don't let that stop me. I regularly travel overseas on business and have visited places as far flung as Sri Lanka and Turkey. On one trip to China, with the help of a few strong friends, I went up the Great Wall. I hate being helped but had to submit to being carried up hundreds of steps. The view from the wall was incredible and it's now one of my favourite memories; the experience taught me to accept help with good grace.

As a young man I wanted to race cars but had limited resources and, if I'm honest, talent. I decided to take up racing a few years after the accident and found it to be an excellent motivator to keeping fit and helped me overcome my shyness about being in a wheelchair. I have now competed in more than 100 races and currently hold an International Race Licence.

After more than two years of testing and development, on 17th September 2008, I set two British Land Speed Records, driving a 1971 Lola T 222 Can-Am Race car. The record attempts were made to demonstrate that significant achievements are not the preserve of the able-bodied. I might have been able to set a few more records, but towards the end of a timed run the car took to the air at over 200mph and somersaulted until it came to rest upside down at the side of the runway. My helmet had come off but I remained conscious. I suffered a number of broken bones and a bump to the head but fortunately no lasting injuries and have since fully recovered.

I have always been driven. If you are going to be successful you have to find something that interests you, you must sustain that interest and it must suit your personality. Then you can excel.

I've set two British Land Speed Records

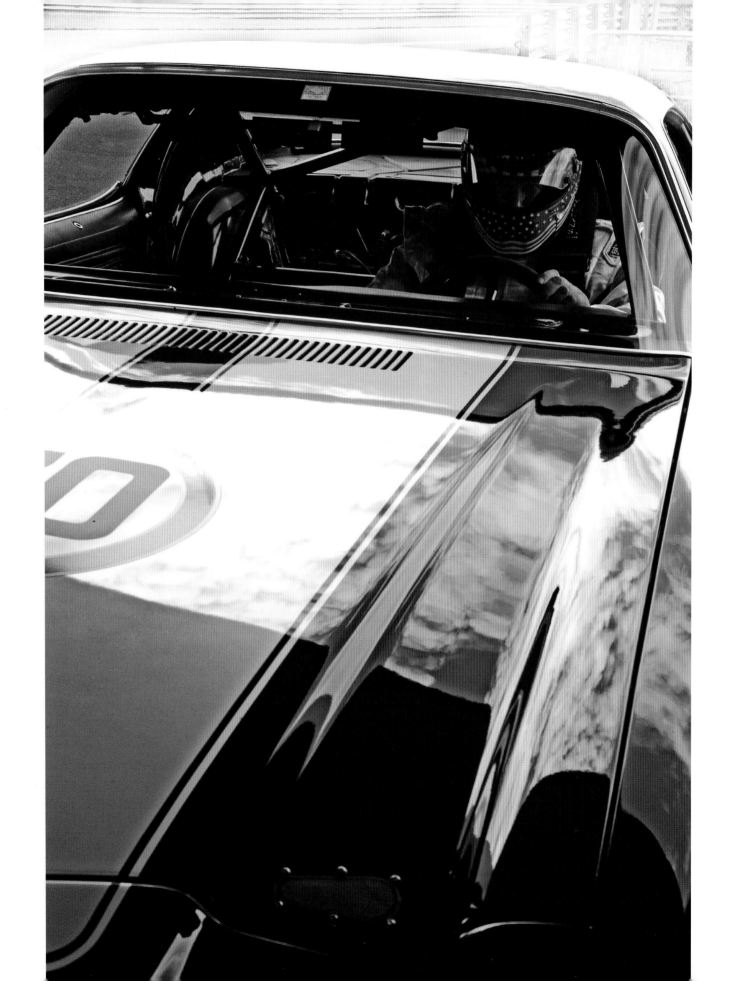

On the 30th May, 2004, my husband, Mark, and I arrived in Australia for the holiday of a lifetime. On the 1st June I became a paraplegic following a horse riding accident.

Before my accident I was a Legal Executive for a firm of solicitors. A typical week would be juggling between preparing cases, attending the Crown Court and also being on 24-hour call for the police station. I was often called out in the middle of the night and expected to be at Court the following day, so life was certainly hectic.

Mark and I liked jive dancing. Following my accident this was probably my biggest loss and something I still have trouble accepting. I find it difficult watching others dance in a way I will never be able to again. Well-meaning people have said I could still dance even though I am in a wheelchair. Sorry, I know they mean well, but it will never be the same and five years further on these wounds are still raw.

Whilst at Stanmore my wonderful husband visited me almost every day, a round trip of 110 miles. One of the hardest times was the first visit home to meet a local occupational therapist; the telephone rang and I automatically tried to get up and answer it. I returned to the hospital with very mixed feelings. There were plenty of 'down days'. The one thought that kept me going was that there was light at the end of the tunnel. I just didn't know how long the tunnel was.

In April 2005 I discovered a great new interest: 10m Air Rifle shooting. I began competing in September 2005 and then entered my first British Open competition in February 2006. I won three gold medals in my class, and since then I have won a variety of medals.

I returned to work, but decided to become self-employed when I became a member of the GB Shooting Team in October 2007. I competed in my first International in December 2007 and achieved three Paralympic minimum qualifying scores. My highest International placing to date is seventh, but I'm working on that.

Life is still hectic, but who would have thought that I would be training for an opportunity at the age of 50 to compete in the Paralympics?

> The telephone rang and I automatically tried to get up and answer it

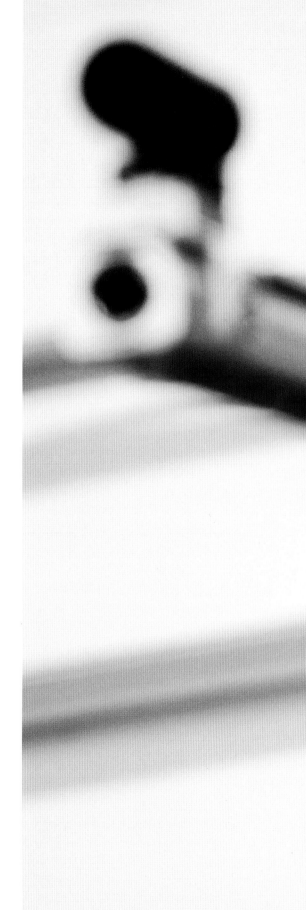

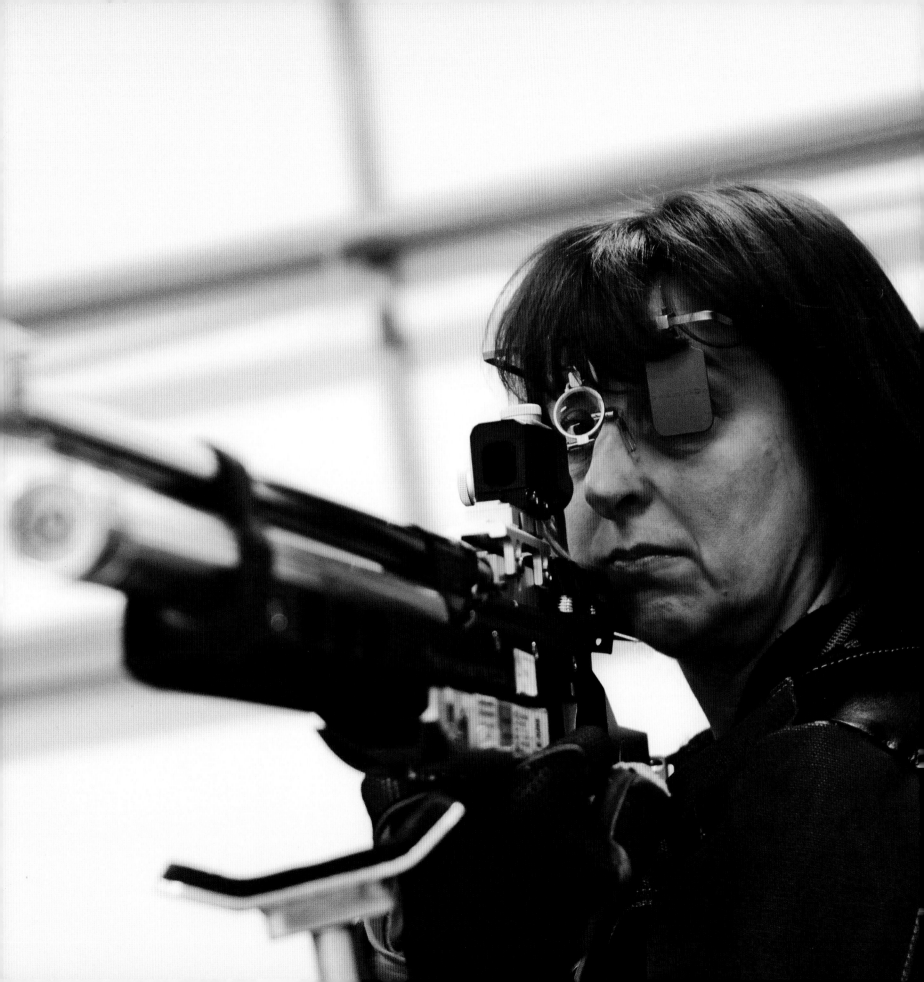

My injury has given me an opportunity to try something I would never have considered before. Some may say "forced me to", but I've always been a glass half-full chap.

For the last six years I have been a busker. My parents put me to the violin at a tender age but it was boring so I gave it up in favour of sports as soon as I could. However, when my legs took early retirement about 15 years ago I had to find a substitute for the sporty stuff, so I tried the violin again and it took.

At first, fiddling was structured therapy. As I improved it became my social life, and in 2003 when busking became legal on the London Underground, I was able to turn my new hobby into a job. I practise every day, work every Friday, Saturday and Sunday for myself, and also busk for a number of charities. I have a regular routine, meet delightful people, feel that I'm making a contribution to society and get money thrown at me. That can't be bad.

I don't do it all by myself, though. Masha, my wife of 50 years, is absolutely essential to the whole enterprise. I try and do what I can around the home, but with my limited mobility that doesn't amount to much. Masha's a wonderful cook, but when it comes to baking our bread I do the 'skillful' bits sitting at the table and she carries the heavy stuff and does the oven thing. On work days, she packs my rucksack on my wheelchair and sees me off the premises. We're a team: that's how we got four sons and eight wonderful grandchildren.

I get grumpy at times, especially at Transport for London's idea of wheelchair accessible buses. Their publicity suggests that London Buses are a wheeler's paradise. Well, they are not, but I am working on it with letters and campaigns.

A spinal cord injury closes some options, but once the daily maintenance tasks are out of the way, the world is still full of opportunities. Like anyone who has come through a life-threatening situation, I have been offered another bite of the cherry. I'm not going to sit around waiting for things to happen. I've been able to indulge a passion for music which I would never have known about. It doesn't have to be music for you, but where there's a passion there's a way.

I'm not going to sit around waiting for things to happen

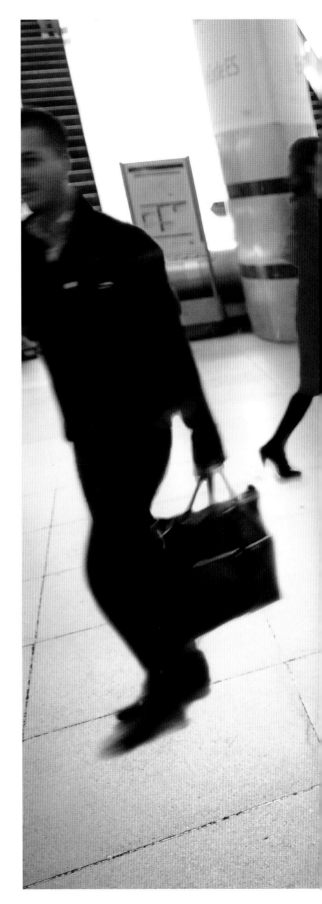

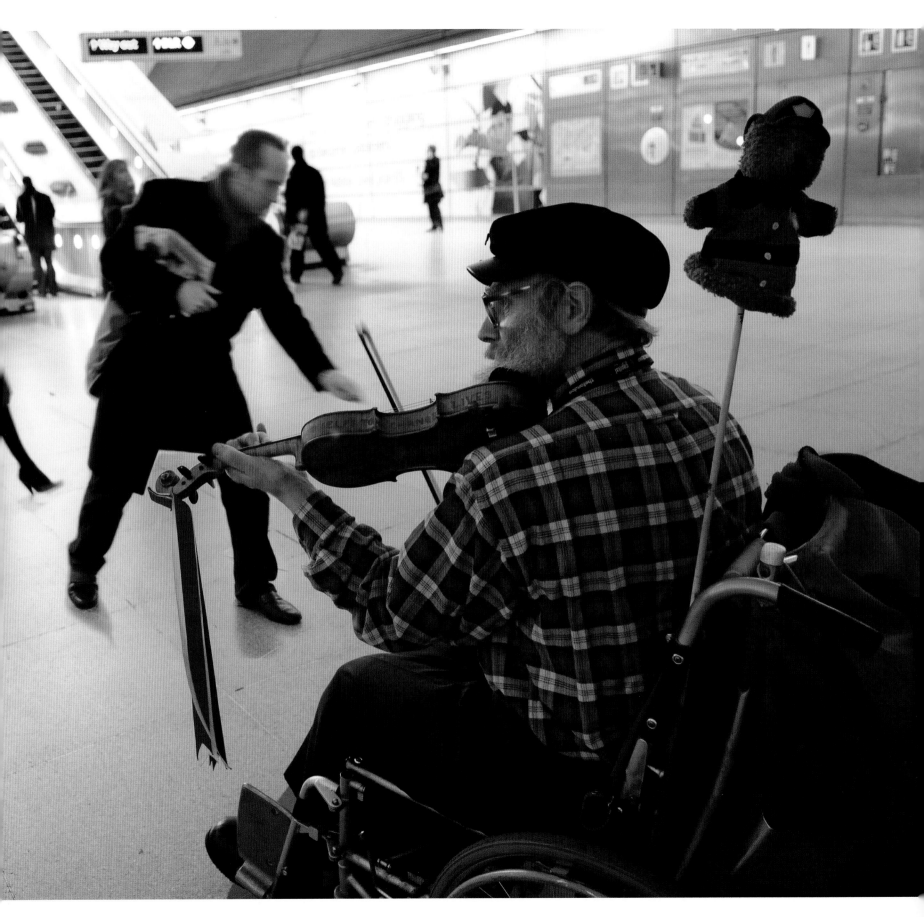

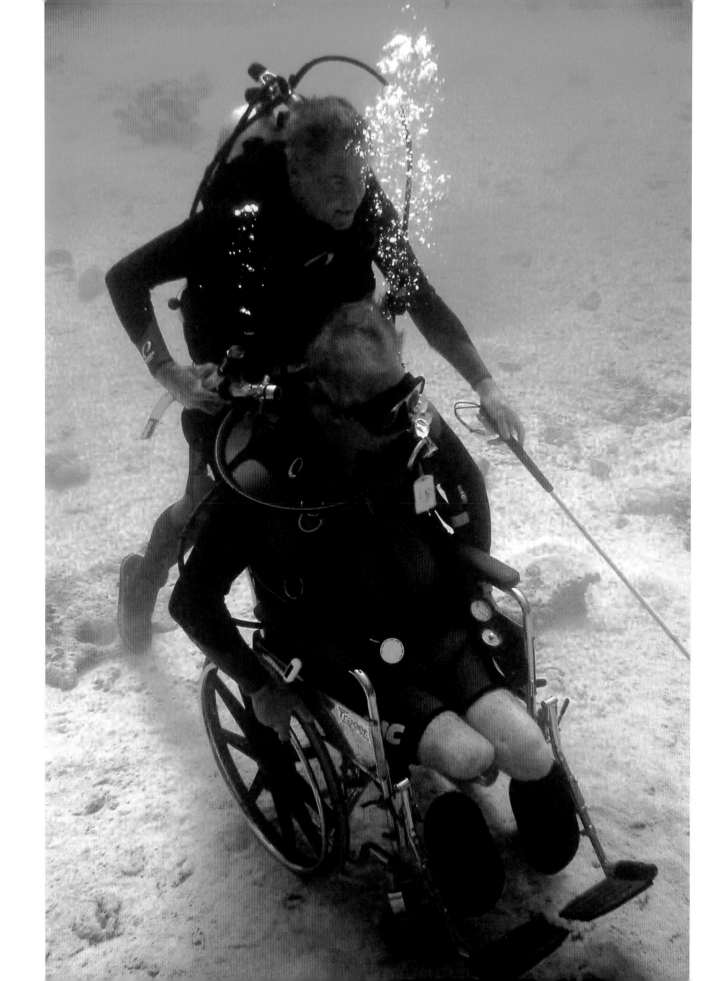

In 1993, I had a bit of a bump while working for an aid agency in Bosnia. After spending a happy 21 years in the wine trade, I had decided to do something completely different and went to work in a war, thinking that this would be more peaceful than selling wine to some restaurateurs, retailers and private individuals. I was very fortunate to survive. Sadly the two people with me were killed.

After about three weeks in an overflow intensive care unit in Split, which I'm told resembled a MASH field hospital, I was airlifted back to London in a coma. One of the advantages of a coma is that it is an easy way to give up smoking as all the withdrawal symptoms happen when you don't know about them. I had tried, unsuccessfully, many ways to give up but this one worked. In total I spent 14 months in hospital.

When you are first aware of what has happened, it is a life-changing experience. To some extent, your previous way of life contributes to how you cope, but I believe luck has something to do with it too. I was fortunate that my brain said, "This is a bit of a bugger but let's get on with it." You can't control your circumstances but you can control your response to them.

This is a bit of a bugger but let's get on with it

Unfortunately, I have spent over five years in hospitals in the last 13, in various stints and many operations. But I've always escaped to more adventures. The biggest so far has been going 'Around the World in 80 Ways' with two blind friends. We achieved 94 different modes of transport in 15 countries over 93 days. I think I may be the only legless paraplegic to have ridden an ostrich, elephant and camel, crashed a balloon and navigated a blind, blonde, Irish girl round a Grand Prix circuit!

Admittedly not as pretty, Miles Hilton Barber, who is also blind but doesn't really need his white stick so many feet under the sea, came up with the idea that we should illustrate that: "The only limits in your life are those you accept yourself". I agreed. I should point out that we are qualified open water divers and normally don't use a stick or chair underwater but a picture of that wouldn't prove a point. You see what we wanted to demonstrate was that if you want to do something enough... you can.

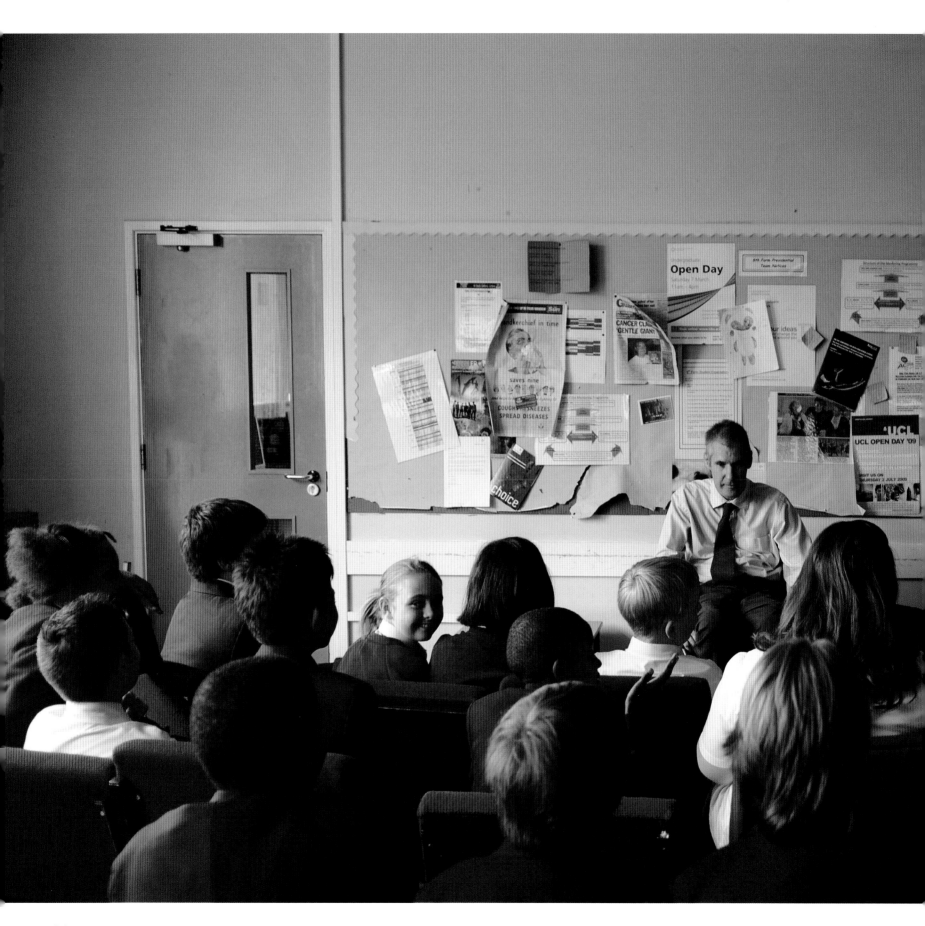

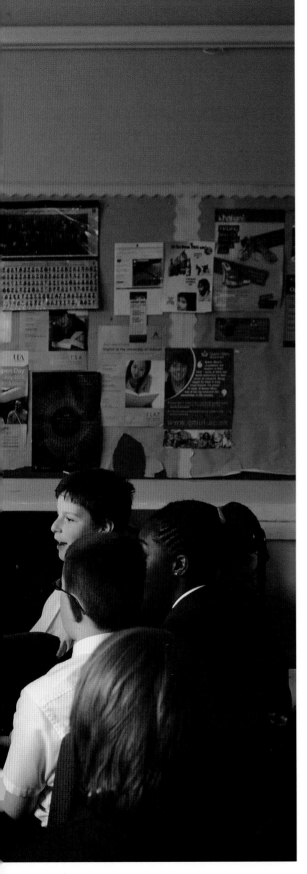

ANDREW'S STORY

Before my injury in 1992 I was Head of PE, but I had to give up that post. Instead, I reverted to my second subject, History, and took on pastoral roles. I still did a little bit of PE teaching from the chair, though. I'm now Head of a Sixth Form.

So many schools are in old buildings and it's not always been easy finding a school that is accessible for me to work in. It has made job hunting rather more difficult over the years. Teaching from a wheelchair is a different experience, but I've managed to adapt with the help of the schools and the students. I feel it is good for them to come into contact with disability first hand. This said, I'm 'Sir' first and a man in a wheelchair second, and they don't offer much in the way of concession.

I'm married to Sarah and have three children. Millie is nearly 17 and from my first marriage. Tom is eight and Jessie seven. I'm truly blessed to have such a wonderful family. I enjoy all sports and spend a lot of time watching my children play sport, or any other sporting events I can get to. I also enjoy reading and socialising.

I despaired a little after my injury, which happened in a road accident, but I got through with the help and support of my friends and family. I also gained massive strength from fellow patients during my time in hospital and from most, if not all, of the other spinally injured people I've met. Seeing others coping with their injuries helped me to get on with it and realise that I was not the only one dealing with all the issues I found myself faced with. The turning point came when I was able to get out of bed and got used to the wheelchair. This was very hard to begin with, much harder than people might think.

I think my friends would describe me as a miserable old git. I'd prefer to describe myself as a wise old sage with a wry take on the world around me. You have to have a sense of humour and perspective when you are confronted with some of the challenges you face in a wheelchair. Being able to laugh at yourself is a tremendous help and puts people at ease when they meet you and your wheels. Falling out of the chair and feigning injury is even better. You get the sympathy vote and they might even give you money…

> # I'm 'Sir' first and a man in a wheelchair second

One of my first memories after my accident is lying in a hospital bed with the slow realisation that something was wrong. I felt frustrated by the slow pace of life in the Spinal Centre and eventually I discharged myself early.

Just over a week after going home, I had an epileptic fit which meant that I lost my driving licence for 12 months. There I was, home alone and unable to drive. Buses and trains were not accessible so I pushed myself everywhere in my wheelchair.

I noticed early on that, when out and about, people would watch me. Although a bit disconcerting, in many ways I was used to this; as a policeman people always gave me a second look and when on my police horse I was often the centre of attention. I persuaded myself that it was just because people were interested that they watched me, not because they thought I looked a freak.

I went back to work and for the first year I was at a local police station answering non-emergency calls. Then I moved up to Scotland Yard answering 999 calls and working on the main radio channels. A change in policy forced me to retire, but luckily I got a job straight away as a civilian doing exactly the same thing. Unfortunately it was for less money.

Whilst still in hospital my thoughts turned to sex or the future lack of it. If I couldn't even walk, how was I going to have sex? No woman would ever be attracted to me. But then I met Susie and we got married. Susie already had three small children and bringing them up would be a challenge for anybody. Surprisingly though, I seem to have found it no harder than anyone else would. At no time has my disability been an issue.

If I had the chance to go back in time, I'd decline

Of course I do miss some things; Susie and I occasionally say how nice it would be to go walking along country tracks rather than pavements and I miss being able to ride my horses like I used to. There have been times I haven't been able to share some things with the family, but these occasions are few and far between and far outweighed by the positive experiences.

I can honestly say that my life has never been better and, if offered the chance to go back in time, I would decline. I simply can't imagine myself being this happy.

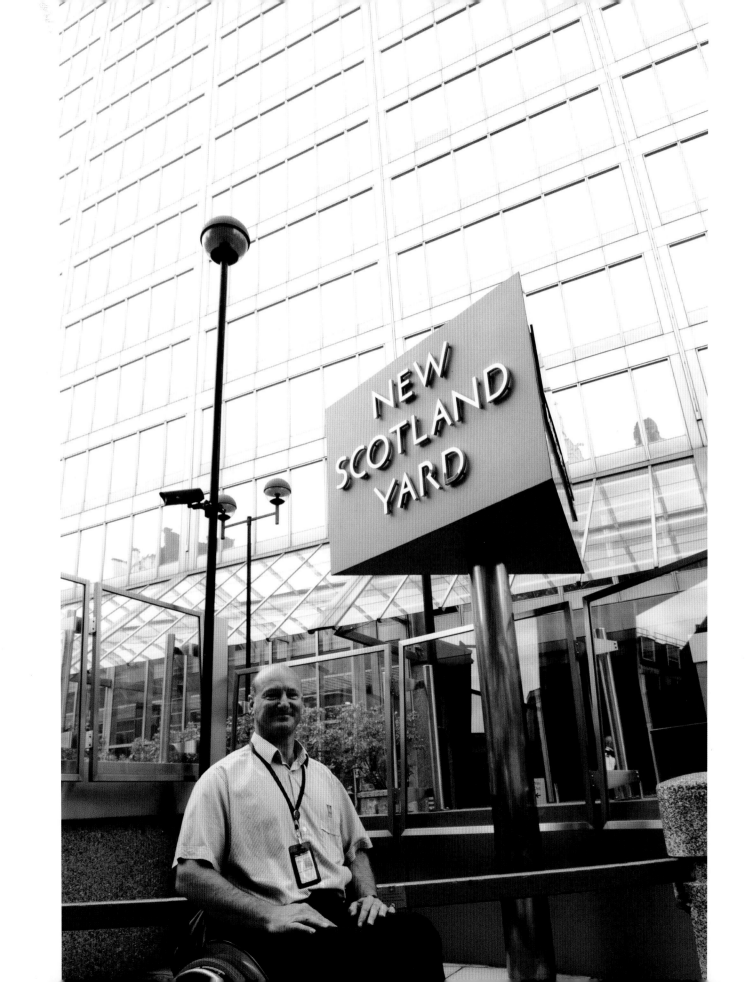

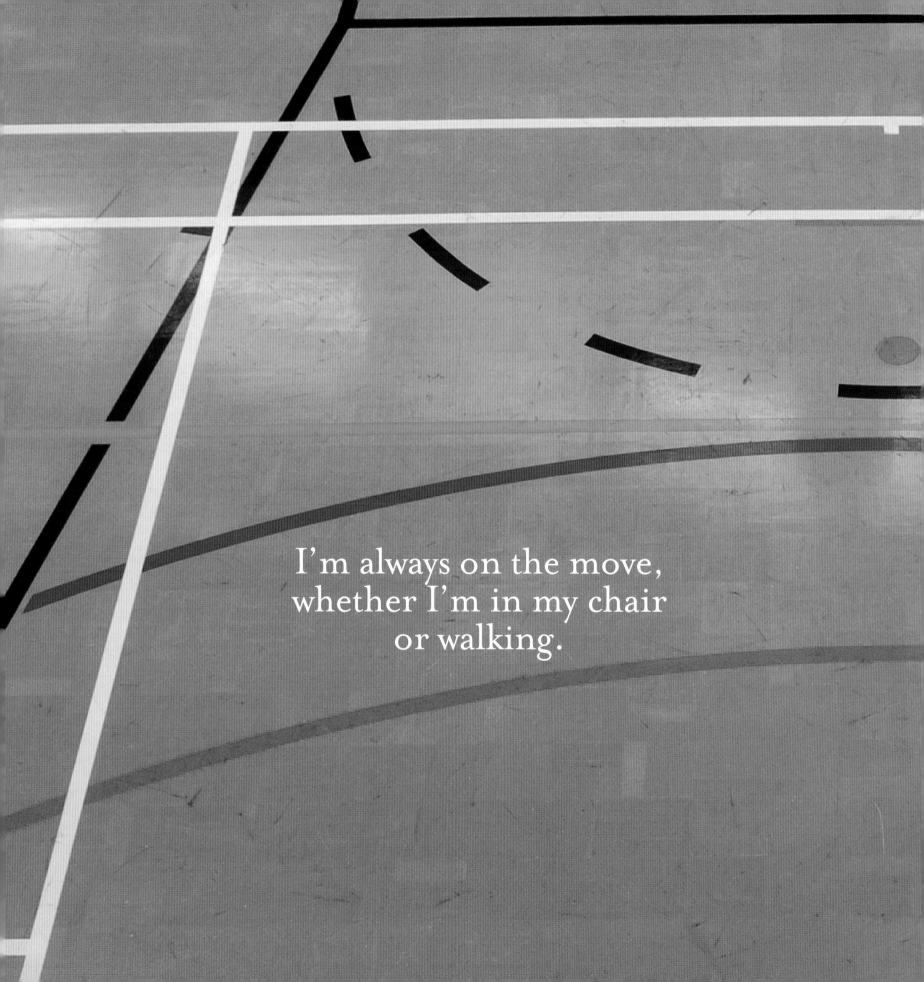

I'm always on the move,
whether I'm in my chair
or walking.

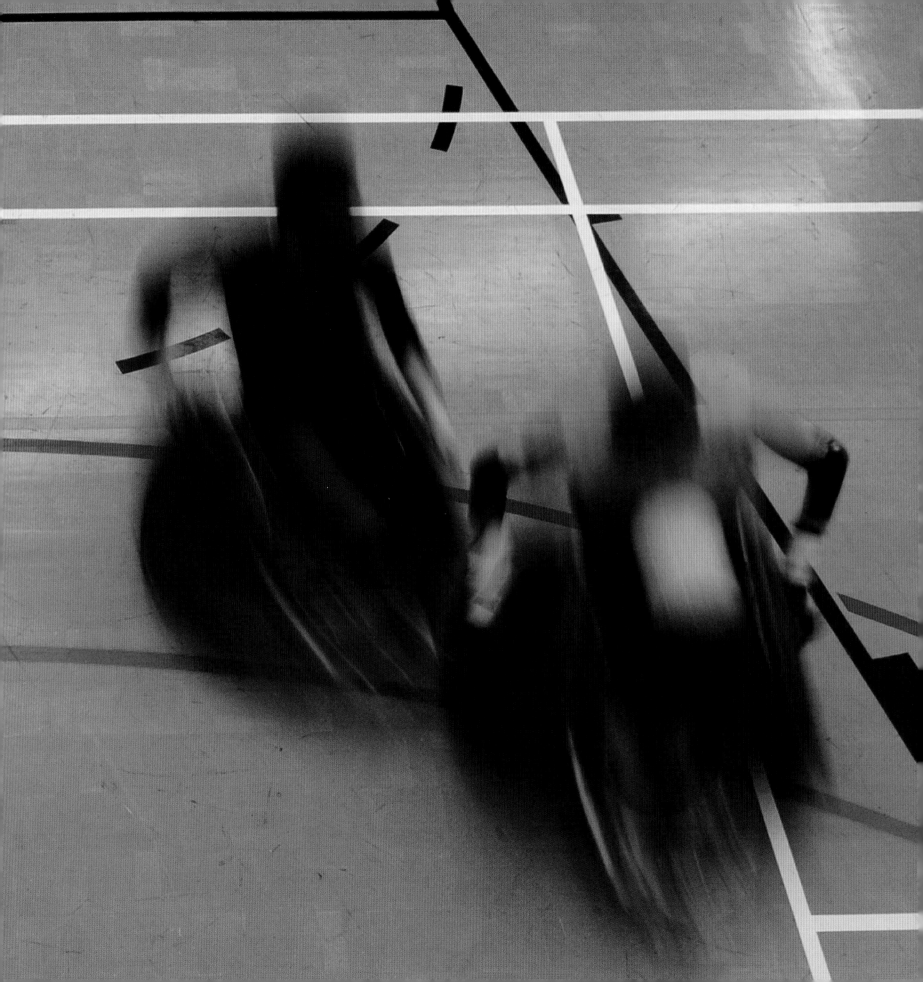

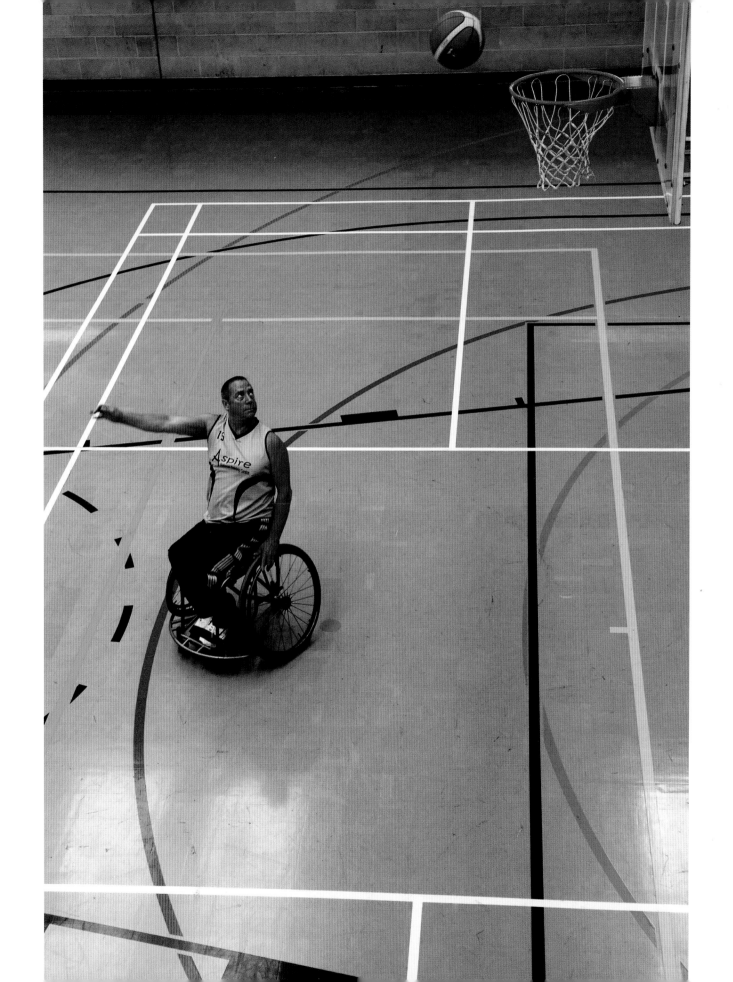

I was determined to walk after I had my accident and I was given full length callipers and crutches. Eventually, I didn't need the crutches and I'm one of the very few spinal breaks I've come across who can walk with callipers but without sticks. I'm always on the move, whether I'm in my chair or walking.

When I got out of hospital it was a bit of a struggle at first to find work. But then I got myself a job selling and maintaining wheelchairs, though it meant that I was travelling thousands of miles around the country every week and seeing little of my family. Around the same time I discovered basketball at Stoke Mandeville, where they were still playing the game in cumbersome old hospital chairs. I thought, 'Hey, looks interesting!' and joined in.

By 1989 I was playing wheelchair basketball for Great Britain and first came across Aspire. They asked me to help them set up a team and Aspire Force was born; I'm immensely proud of the fact that the ladies', junior and men's teams have played every Saturday since. Chairs have improved immeasurably in that time, which hopefully will mean less wear and tear on the body for the players in years to come. Of course, I still play and coach whenever I get the chance, too.

Now that I'm working full-time at Aspire as their maintenance manager, I get to talk to lots of patients who come here. I tell them that really their life begins when they leave the hospital, go home and are on their own. My main problems are pain, sores and bladder issues. Poorly fitting and heavy wheelchairs and ageing haven't helped. Both shoulders have been dislocated and I have arthritis in my knees. Years ago, I even leant against a hot fireguard, smelled burning and had to make a mad dash to the hospital. It took weeks to heal.

Some days I feel low, and then I think how lucky I am. I have travelled all round the world playing basketball, met and married my first wife and had two lovely kids. Sadly, she died a few years ago but I've been really fortunate in marrying again. If I had a wish for a day, I'd reverse things and put the able-bodied in a chair and give the wheelchair users a day of walking and running about and dancing.

> # Some days I feel low, and then I think how lucky I am

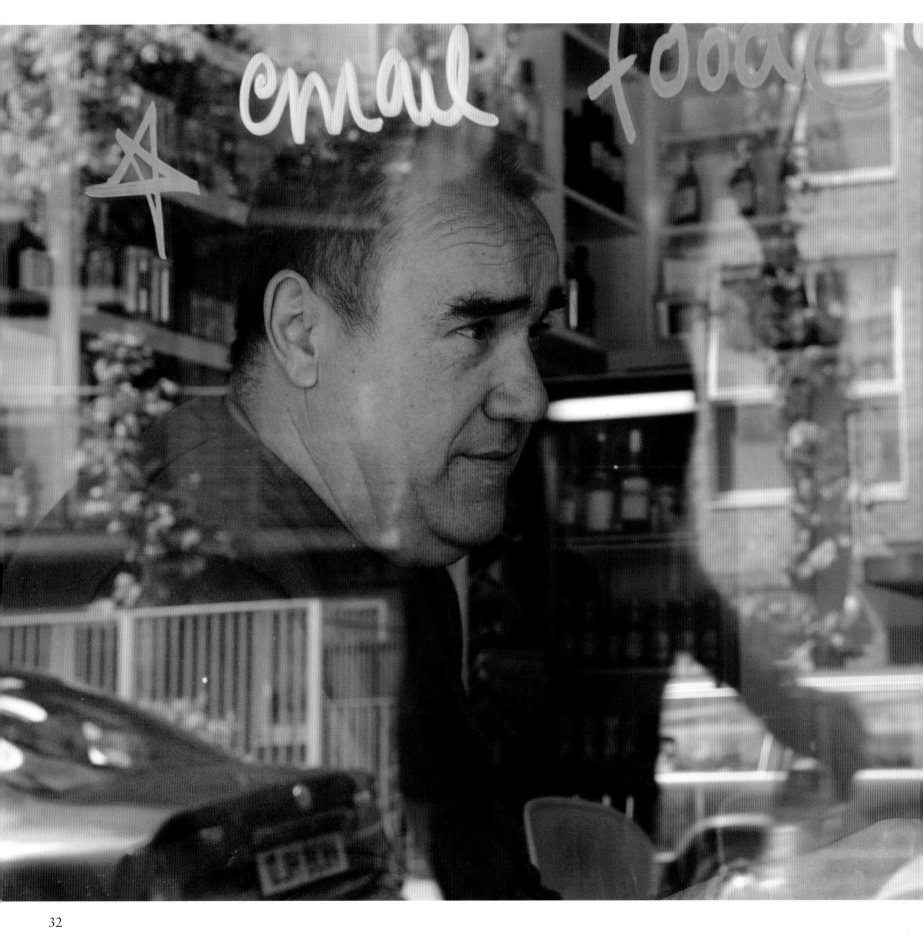

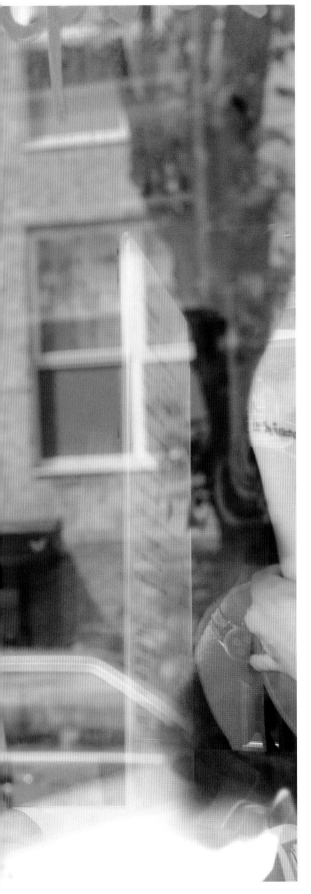

I was a regular at Aspire's National Training Centre for many years, playing wheelchair rugby with the London Broncos, now the London Wheelchair Rugby Club, and travelling on several European tours. I'm pleased to say the club is now number one in Europe. There were only about seven of us playing when I started in London. Now there are dozens all over the country.

I became tetraplegic at 17 following a skiing accident. I had my rehab in a brilliant spinal unit in Geneva; the doctor in charge of the unit was a paraplegic, so I knew there was life after spinal injury.

Although my pre-injury life centred on sport (my favourites were skiing, rugby and boxing), I managed to scrape into Oxford where I stayed for ages, finally leaving in 1982 with a couple of degrees.

When I finally dragged myself away from academic life, which had mostly comprised of loafing around and drinking, I discovered, to my shock, that I had become a social worker. It was temporary. Within a short time, I moved to London where somebody kindly appointed me director of a disability arts company. I also got to make a few documentaries for the newly formed Channel 4. Around this time, I became actively involved in disability politics.

And then I needed a change. So I moved to San Francisco where I'd found a job running a medical research foundation. The access was a revelation. Unlike in London, there was almost no place I could not get into. Due to the lack of physical barriers, I felt much less disabled living in the US than in the UK.

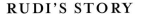

But I'm still looking

I returned to London and went back into television. In the late 1990s I took up playing wheelchair rugby full-time. The new millennium brought with it a diversity of new roles, including as a life coach. When I turned 50, I more or less lost the plot entirely and emigrated to Costa Rica. That didn't work out either. But I'm still looking.

So: what have I learnt? Well, although there's a lot that's tough about being in a wheelchair, it's perfectly possible to lead a rich and varied life if you're prepared to look for it. Don't let your disability lead you to say, "I can't", when you can say, "I can". It takes some work and application but the payback is that the quality of your life will be hugely improved. Just don't hold back.

I started working for a lift company when I was 19, and within a few years was a fully qualified engineer. Having worked at various places, I started my own company which did really well. We were so busy that I had to stop working in the field and help run the business from the office.

My last day on the road saw me at a restaurant where the dumb waiter had broken. I was just starting to investigate the problem when it lost traction and pulled me down the shaft with it. I fell three floors.

I spent time in intensive care, and then many boring weeks on the spinal unit. When I asked to meet someone who had had their spinal injury for a while and could act as a mentor I was introduced to a chap injured in the process of burgling a house, not exactly the role model and motivation to return to work I was looking for!

When I was eventually fit enough, a couple of nurses helped me into a huge NHS wheelchair. They meant well, but I was totally devastated and left wondering how on earth I was going to ever get around. Another chap stopped by and asked if I was OK; he was wheeling himself to his car at the time and, though it sounds strange now, I asked if I could watch him and see how he got himself and the chair into it. From that moment on I was away, I knew I could go wherever I wanted. The future was going to be different, but it was going to be OK.

Since my injury I've continued to build up my company, become an advanced scuba diver and flown an aeroplane. My wife Amanda and I have travelled the world together, always with a smile and an open mind. We've had some great times.

The future was going to be different, but it was going to be OK

I never give up hope that one day I will walk again and I've been a guinea pig a few times with some experimental and painful, but sadly unsuccessful, operations in an attempt to repair my spinal cord.

My advice would be not to believe everything you hear on the ward. Oh, and don't let anyone alter your house until you've tried living in it - I've got a lavatory I need a ladder to reach! Unfortunately, people will stare at you, especially when you're getting in and out of a car. I usually tell them, "I do it a lot quicker in the rain!"

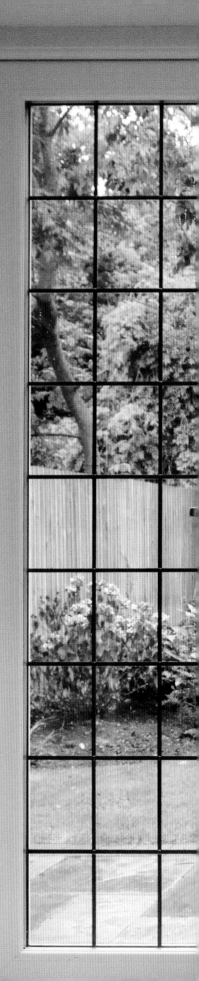

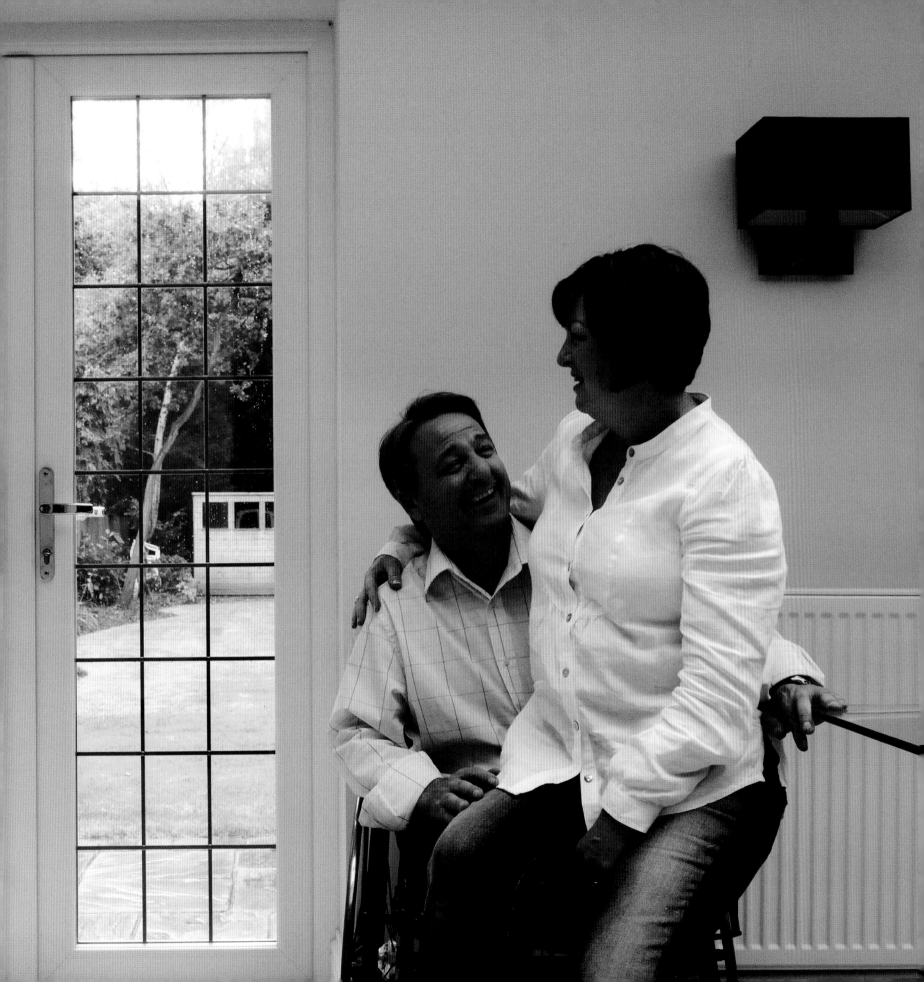

I had been a Detective Constable for nine years when I had my accident. I had previously been a radiographer at St Thomas' Hospital in London but had always wanted to be a policewoman. I wanted to do something different every day.

I am now a Detective Inspector on a Murder Investigation Team having been promoted twice since my accident. My injury rarely gets in the way at work. If I'm visiting somewhere inaccessible, I can always ask someone to lift me up some steps. I am not trained to use a firearm but I am trained to supervise firearms operations, if it is ever required.

Sport has always been important to me. I ran the London Marathon for six consecutive years, 1995 to 2000. In 2000, I ran in 2 hours and 57 minutes and then, in 2002, following my accident, I competed in the women's wheelchair race. In 2004, I came second in 2 hours and 6 minutes.

In 2001, I was out on my bike, training for a triathlon, when I was hit by a car driven by a very old man who just didn't see me. I still compete in triathlons and training takes up a lot of my free time. I sometimes work long hours and I am also the sports governor at Amwell View School which is a school for children and young people with special needs. There never seem to be enough hours in the day to do all I would like to do.

As an athlete, I draw inspiration from Sir Steve Redgrave. The thought of him getting up so early for all those years to train at that level is amazing, especially with his own health issues. I also draw inspiration from my own family and friends, everyone has their own problems. I read recently that if everyone threw their problems into a pile, we would still choose to take our own back. I think that is so true.

My family is Catholic and we all have this great faith to draw on in times of trouble. The serenity prayer, which includes 'grant me the serenity to accept the things I cannot change; courage to change the things I can; and wisdom to know the difference' is one I use a lot.

Shortly after my accident, someone said to my brother, "I'm sorry to hear about Paula; her life is over now really, isn't it?" Thankfully, he said, "You'd better try telling her that!"

My injury rarely gets in the way at work

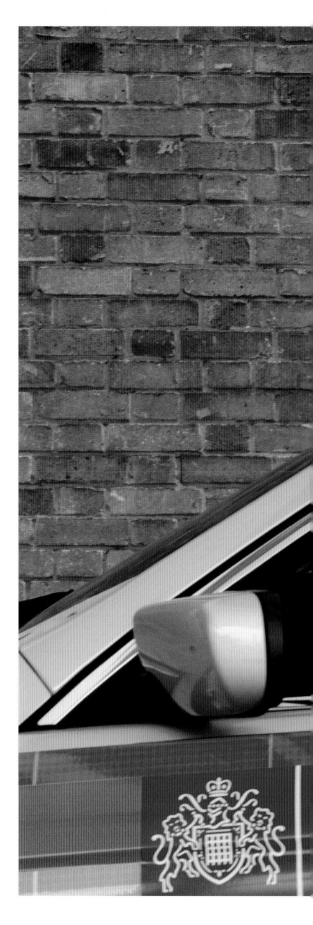

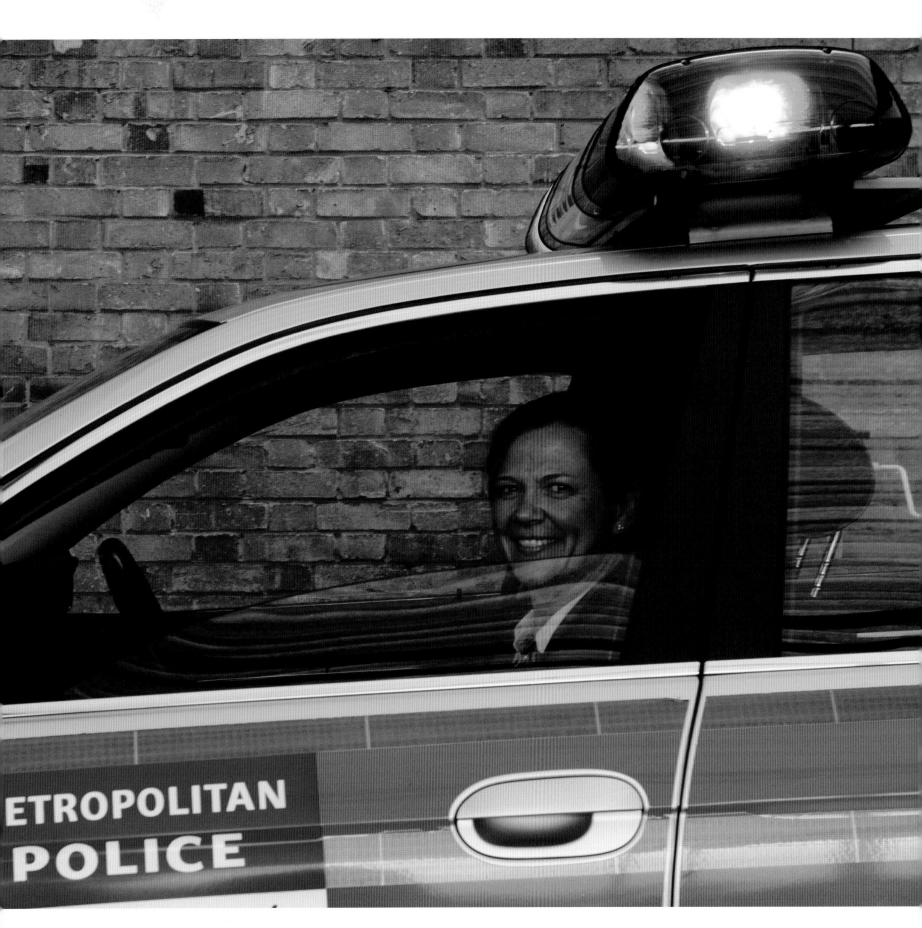

ETROPOLITAN
POLICE

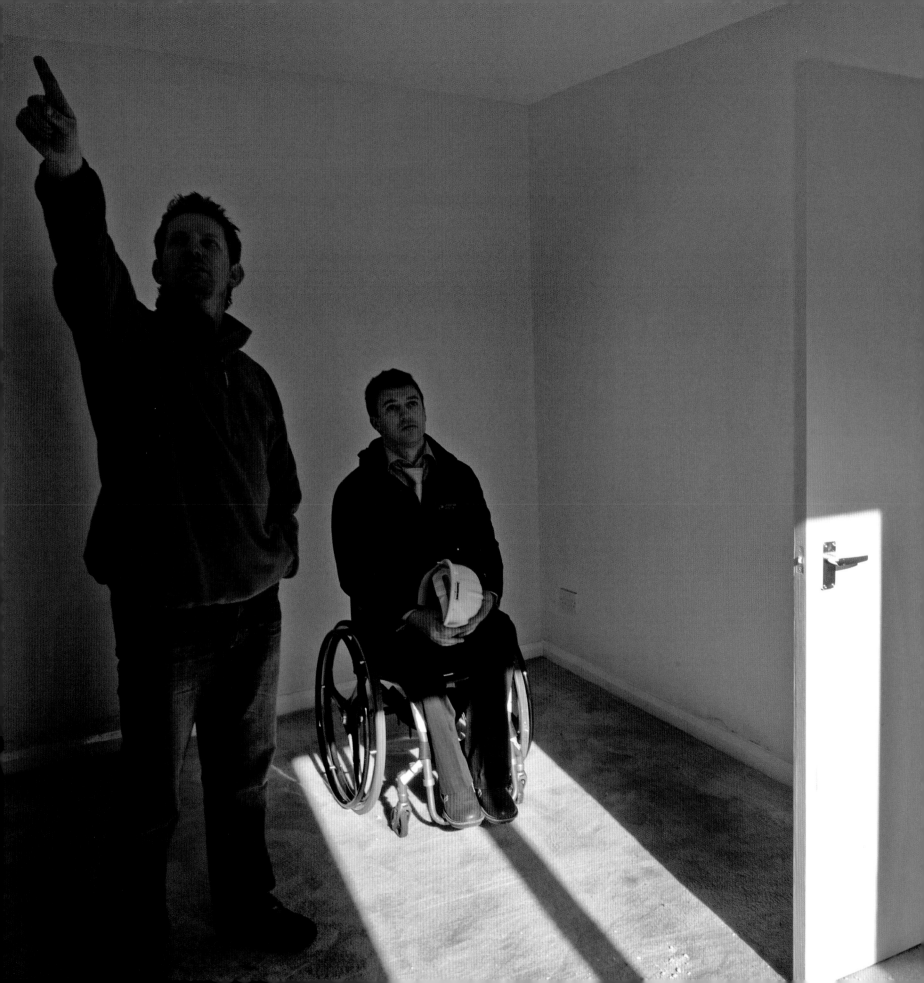

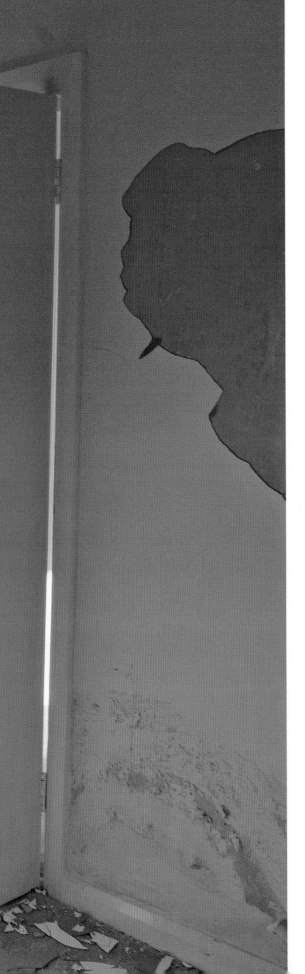

LUKE'S STORY

I used to feel sorry for people in wheelchairs. I used to wonder how they could enjoy their lives when they looked so different. Then, two weeks before my 18th birthday, I was injured in a road traffic accident. One minute I was planning to go around the world travelling, the next I was in a spinal injuries unit, feeling my life was never going to be the same again.

However, I was still looking out of the same pair of eyes and the world looked exactly the same as it had before my accident. Catching sight of myself in the mirror was a bit of a shock at first – there I was as the sort of person I used to feel sorry for.

For many years I assumed all people had the same feelings I'd had about wheelchair-users. So if they offered me help, it was only because they felt sorry for me and thought I had a pretty sad life. Looking back, it's funny now to remember how I used to feel annoyed that people had dared to notice my wheelchair. How could they miss it?! Now I realise people just want to connect with other people, and offering help is completely instinctive. Seeing this has been the most liberating experience of my life.

I look at the things I can do and not at the things I can't. I've had amazing relationships, and only one girl has said she would never go out with someone in a wheelchair again; she didn't like the attention it caused when we were out. Believe it or not, I've found being in a chair can be an advantage when it comes to going up and meeting new people, although I've still embarrassed myself countless times! When it comes to sex, okay, I can't stand up, and I don't have much hip movement, but I've had very few complaints, so I must be doing something right!

It's now seventeen years since my accident and life has continued to be good. I have worked in the City and in television, playing long-running characters in *The Bill* and *Casualty*, and I've run my own property lettings business. With so much going on, it's rare not to have something needing to be done or somewhere to be but if I have a down time, I get out into the fresh air, go to the gym or ring a mate.

It's still a shock when I see another wheelchair user in my part of town, though - I like to think of myself as the only chair in the village!

> # The world looks exactly the same as it did before

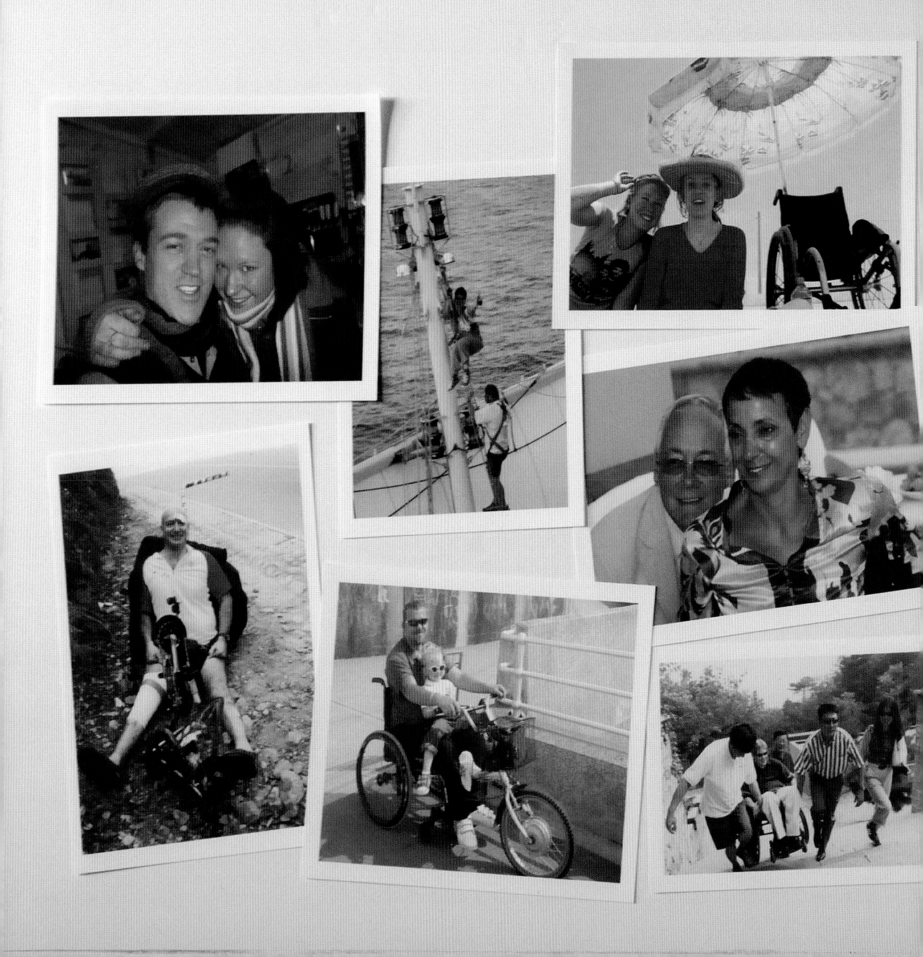

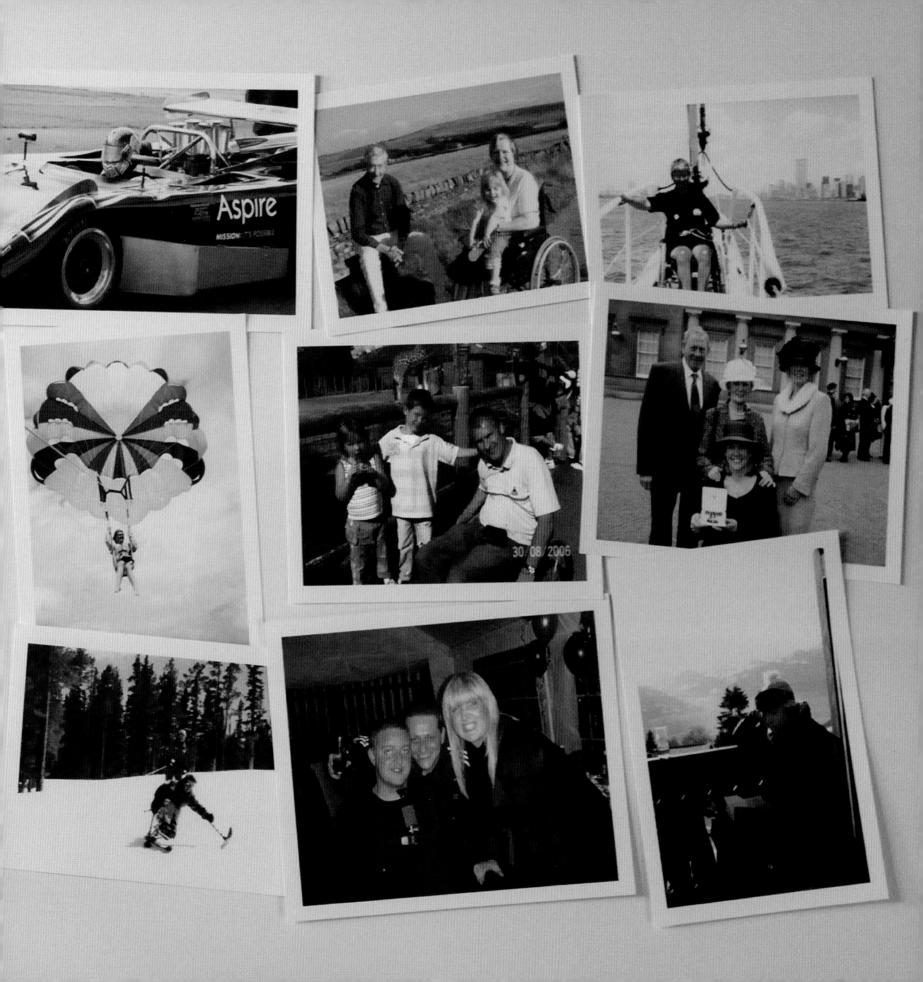

Two days after the motorbike accident I woke up with my girlfriend holding my hand and telling me I had to fight as she was pregnant. I left the Spinal Centre just in time to be there for the birth of our daughter, Lilly-Ann.

Times were difficult at first, but when my wife returned to work as a primary-school teacher we decided that I would stay at home and look after Lilly-Ann. It was daunting, but she was what had kept me going for the past year, and I was definitely up for the challenge. I might not have as much time for the gym as before, what with Lilly-Ann and the school pick-ups coming before anything else, but it's all good.

Before the accident I had been in the garage trade for 15 years, but I found it difficult to go back to it. Instead, I decided to retrain as a web designer and go to university – it was all really different as, even now, I'm still not used to sitting about in one place for too long. The old skills aren't completely lost, though, and my newest project is to build a trike, based on a VW Beetle. There's nothing like the wind in your face and bugs in your teeth to make it all worthwhile! I have a good friend who is also in a wheelchair and into his trikes so, when it's done, we're planning on travelling around the UK together and visiting the various Spinal Centres.

I've been told that I'm a bit of a 'Victor Meldrew' character. I have built and designed a website, www.space-d-out.co.uk, that allows people who get fed up with non-disabled people abusing disabled parking bays to name and shame the culprits. I've heard all sorts of excuses from perpetrators at the local supermarket and shops, and had some abuse for challenging those who shouldn't be using the bays. It's just one of the irritating issues anyone with a disability experiences every day and you get used to it. You don't have to like it, though, and the website is my way of dealing with it.

My physio and I are currently embarking on a new challenge to see if I can use back-slabs and, hopefully, move on to callipers. It might not be enough to walk properly, but I would be able to stand and sit at the cinema or restaurants with my wife and daughter and mates like anyone else. That would mean the world to me.

> # I've been told that I'm a bit of a Victor Meldrew

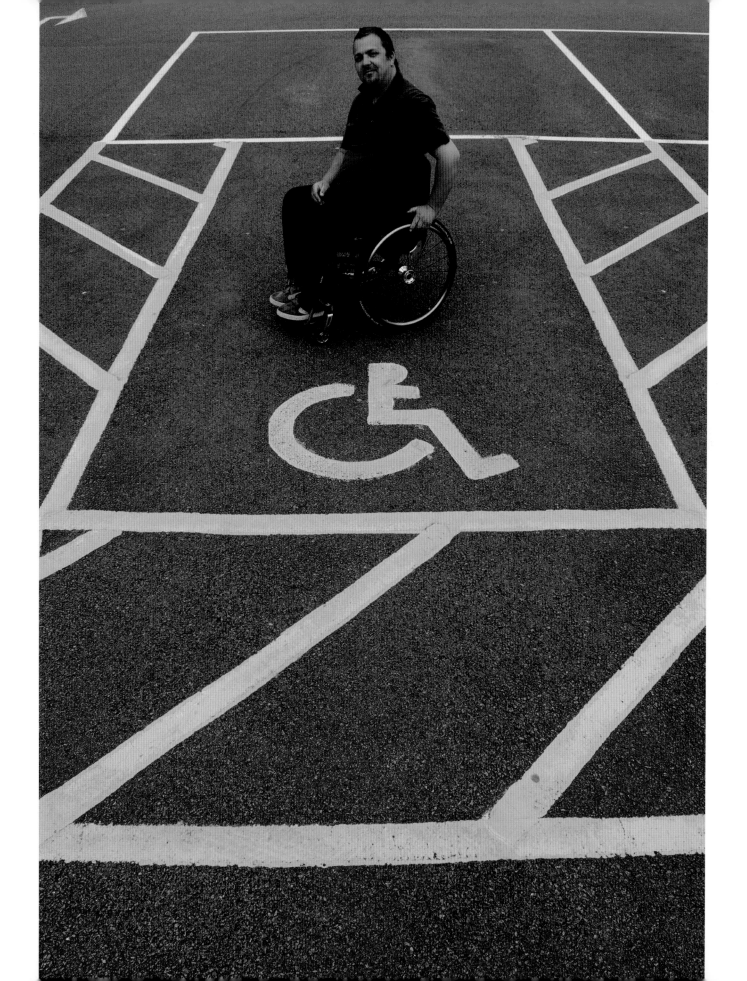

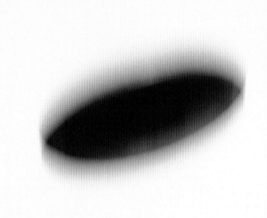

After my accident I was very low. If someone had given me a pill, I would have taken it there and then. If I had, I would never have travelled the world, had my wonderful children, met the Queen, visited Downing Street and had Eamonn Andrews present me with a *This is your Life* book. And I would never have won a Paralympic gold medal for Great Britain in discus throwing - a world record of 32 metres and 82 centimetres.

I thought I'd be an international playboy

When I was 18 I fell 40 feet onto a wall from the big wheel at a fairground in Minehead. To begin with, when I was leaving the unit, I thought I'd be an international playboy. I had always had this idea about myself that I was invincible, some sort of Superman. The local job centre had other ideas. They actually came round to my house to make sure I got out of bed and out of doors, and they tried very hard to find a vocation for me. But in Wales, back then, it was just the steel works, the coal mines or driving a coal lorry.

It wasn't easy and for the first three years I just went down to the pub and drank, smoked and went home and slept. My dad had died when I was young so my mum was my life. One day, she said: "You've got to start changing. One day you won't have any friends and I will have gone and you'll be all on your own." That scared me, and then I met a chap in the pub who suggested I should go with him down to my local sports centre. Six weeks later, I was ready to join a body-building club. After that, it was like a domino effect, with one thing following another; I took part in a multi-sport competition and won everything I entered, then joined a club that did field events. Soon I was taking part in the internationals.

I have a smashing family and love spending time with my kids. For some reason I have always got on well with young people, there is something about a wheelchair that interests them. Very young kids can talk to you easily; after all, you're not very high up.

I think you've just got to accept what you've got and don't look to walking up the street. Get to like yourself as you are. Be positive, dream your dreams and give people a smile as you go along. Forty-five years on, I'm still dreaming but I wouldn't change my life, not one bit of it.

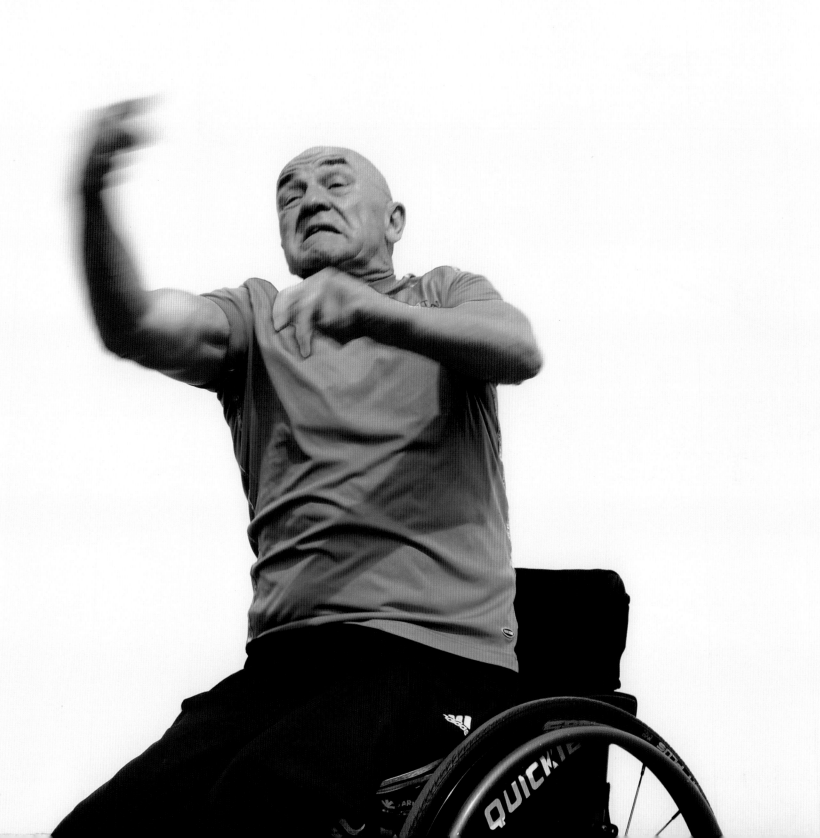

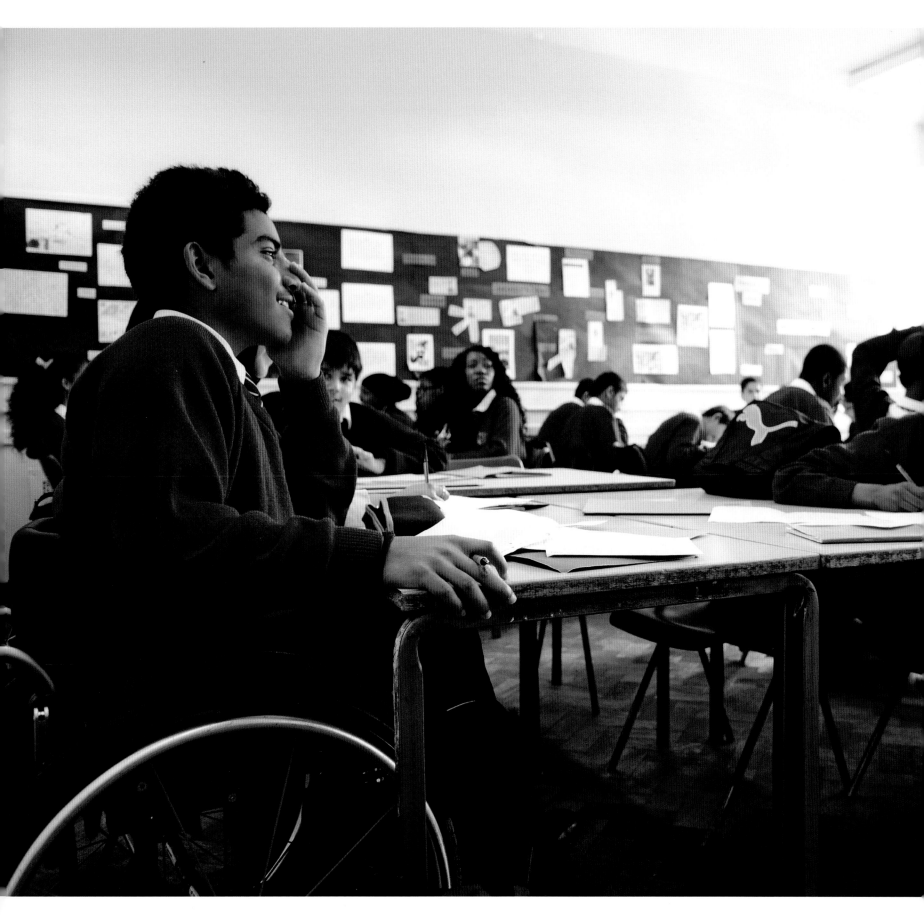

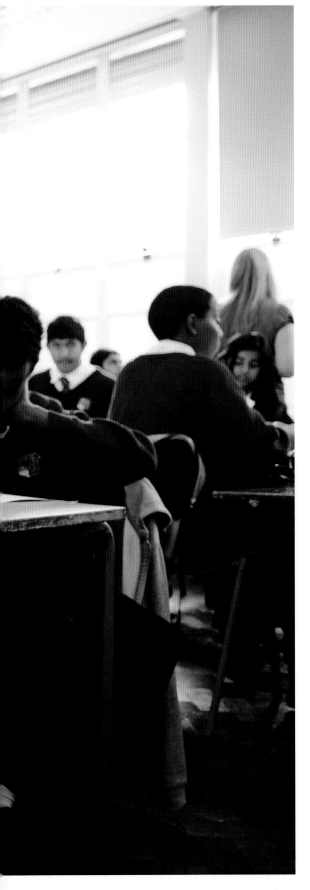

SHEIKE'S STORY

I'm 13, and I think my friends would probably describe me as energetic, friendly and cheeky.

I am hoping to do swimming or wheelchair racing at the 2012 Paralympics in London. At the moment I am concentrating on choosing between them, and then I can really train properly. I love all sports. I play basketball and have won lots of medals at the Stoke Mandeville games. And I've done the London mini marathon three times, and lots of other wheelchair events too. Sometimes people stop me in the street to congratulate me, usually because they have seen a story about me winning in the local newspaper. Their interest really encourages me to keep up with my sports.

When I was six and a half years old, I was hit by a car when I was crossing the road. I don't remember anything about it. I thought that afterwards I would not have a life like other children and I was sad.

After my accident in Kenya, my family encouraged me not to lose hope. After that I started to work towards being independent. It was hard at first. I was in a lot of pain and used not to sleep at night, especially when it became severe and I went through a period where I thought life was not worth it, but now I am happy. With my family's support, I have learned to cope.

My mum used to have to carry me, but some time after my accident people made a collection to buy me a wheelchair. After that life started to become easier. A few years ago my parents and I came to England and I went to a special school. Everyone was really kind and I made some friends, but now I go to a regular secondary school and I really enjoy learning. I especially like maths and anything that's challenging; it keeps me alive. I don't have problems with people at school; they open doors for me and they tell me they like my wheels.

When I am grown up, I hope to have a Lamborghini, a black or red one with a spoiler and 20 inch alloy wheels. My only advice to anyone with a spinal cord injury is please don't give up. Keep on trying and you will get what you want. Don't think negative thoughts.

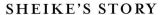

They tell me they like my wheels, but I want a Lamborghini

Before my injury I worked as a Graphic Designer, but the studio where I worked could not be made wheelchair accessible. Also, because of physical challenges such as severe spasms and incontinence, it took a few years before I felt ready to resume work.

Since 2007, I've worked as a VJ in nightclubs: this involves playing and projecting video clips that work in rhythm with music played by a DJ or live band. I love this work because it combines music with art in a very immediate way. I get lots of positive feedback, although occasionally I do get mistaken for the DJ!

My part-time day job is helping to run the Mystery Shopping project for Attitude is Everything, an organisation committed to improving disabled access in the UK music industry. I also do occasional work as a freelance journalist, and voluntary work for SGI-UK, a Buddhist organisation dedicated to world peace. In my free time, I enjoy going to parties, gigs, and festivals, both here and abroad. So far this year, the most fun I've had was at dance music festival, the Glade, in southern England. Meanwhile, back in London, my favourite party was Tru Playaz Carnival Special, at Fabric, where I danced all night to the best drum & bass I'd heard in ages.

Although some of the staff were very supportive, I still hated being in hospital. However, my Buddhist practice, and the support of friends and family, helped me become a lot more positive. Also, staying in an Aspire bungalow rather than having to

I was back in control of my life

live in another institution upon discharge helped enormously. It was a place where friends and family could stay the night, and I was back in control of my life.

The real turning point for me happened when, a year after discharge, my boyfriend left me. I realised I had been too dependent on him for help with everything. Having to deal with things on my own made me stronger.

Immediately after injury, the doctors on the spinal unit told me that I'd never walk again, but I've never really accepted that. I do exercises to help 'wake up' my paralysed muscles, and I'm also hopeful of advances in stem cell research. However, I do accept that right now I am paralysed and a full-time wheelchair user, and that I must make the best of this situation.

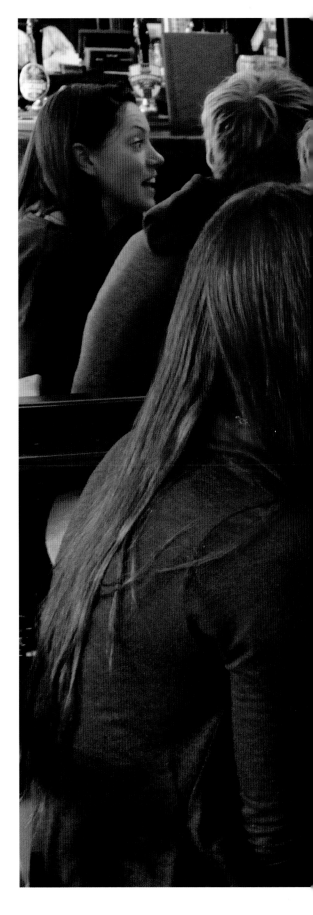

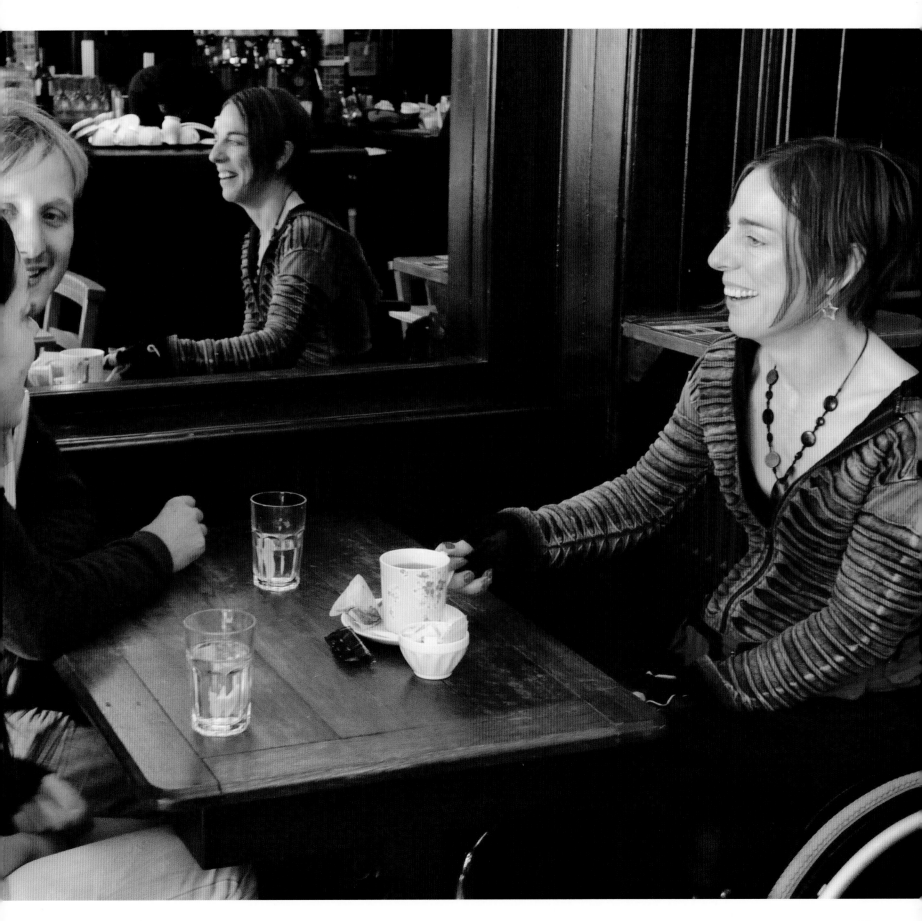

I was 21 when I was injured and totally ignorant about disability. While I was still a patient at my spinal injuries centre, my cousin and his wife, who are great friends, suggested I go and spend a few days with them. Their house is large and my cousin is big and strong so he could carry me upstairs. I went for four days. It was great to be out of hospital, but it made me see how much I had to learn in order to be independent.

I've moved six times since my injury. At first I returned to my parents' house in Sussex, and later moved into a house I shared with my brother. Three years later I moved to London but I had great difficulties finding a suitable place to buy. I ended up renting a flat in a warden-controlled housing scheme for a year, but then could not renew the tenancy. I had no choice but to go and live in a bedsit in an old people's home for over six months; that was dire. Luckily I had a job to go to each day, and I went out as much as possible in the evenings. It was only the knowledge that I would be moving out as soon as the building works were finished on my new flat that kept me sane.

Eventually I moved into a lovely ground floor flat and was there until I came to my current house, a converted cow-shed in a small village just outside Oxford. I hope that this will be my last move, as I am very happy here.

Although a qualified solicitor, I prefer to have more direct contact with clients so I work with other lawyers in my firm and provide additional support to our clients. I help them claim the correct benefits, find suitable housing, choose a wheelchair, locate a driving assessment centre and get cars adapted or buy new ones. I suspect my career has been more varied and possibly more interesting than it would have been had I not been injured. My injury has certainly given me a direction and motivation that I did not have before.

I love cooking and entertaining. I enjoy going to the theatre and occasionally to concerts. I sing in a local choral society, and in the summer I sail a Challenger, a one-man trimaran, competing in local sailing club race nights and at Challenger regattas. In late 2006, I sailed across the Atlantic in a tall ship, which was an amazing experience.

I had so much to learn to be independent

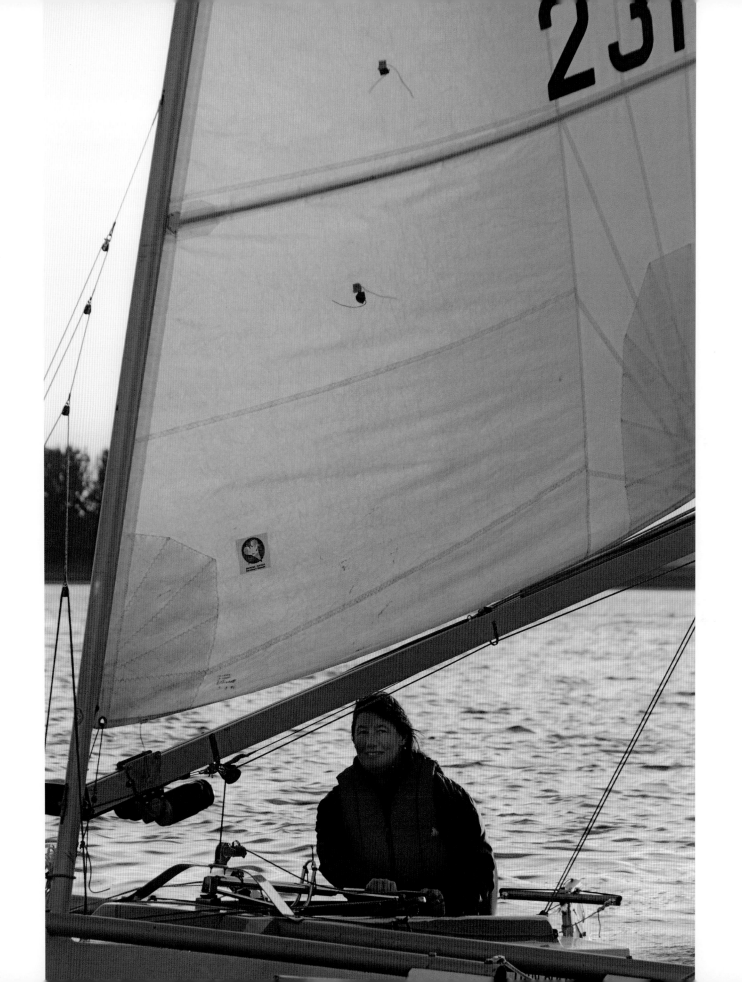

We were creative
and pushed the
boundaries.

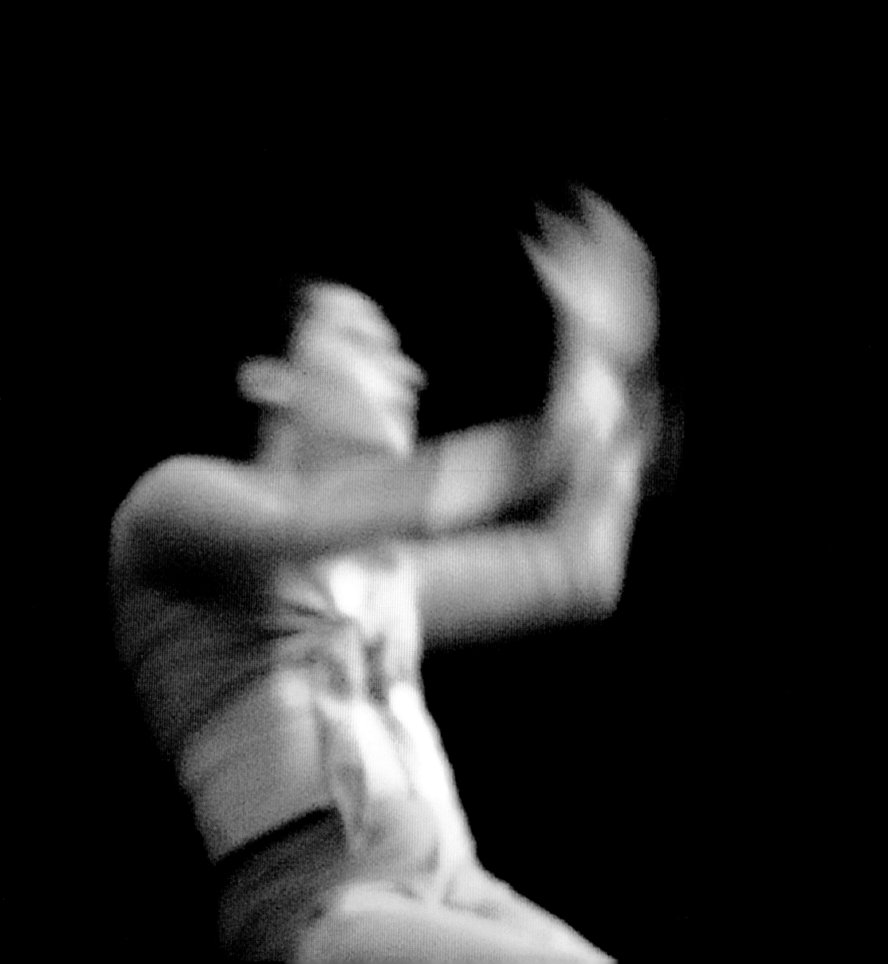

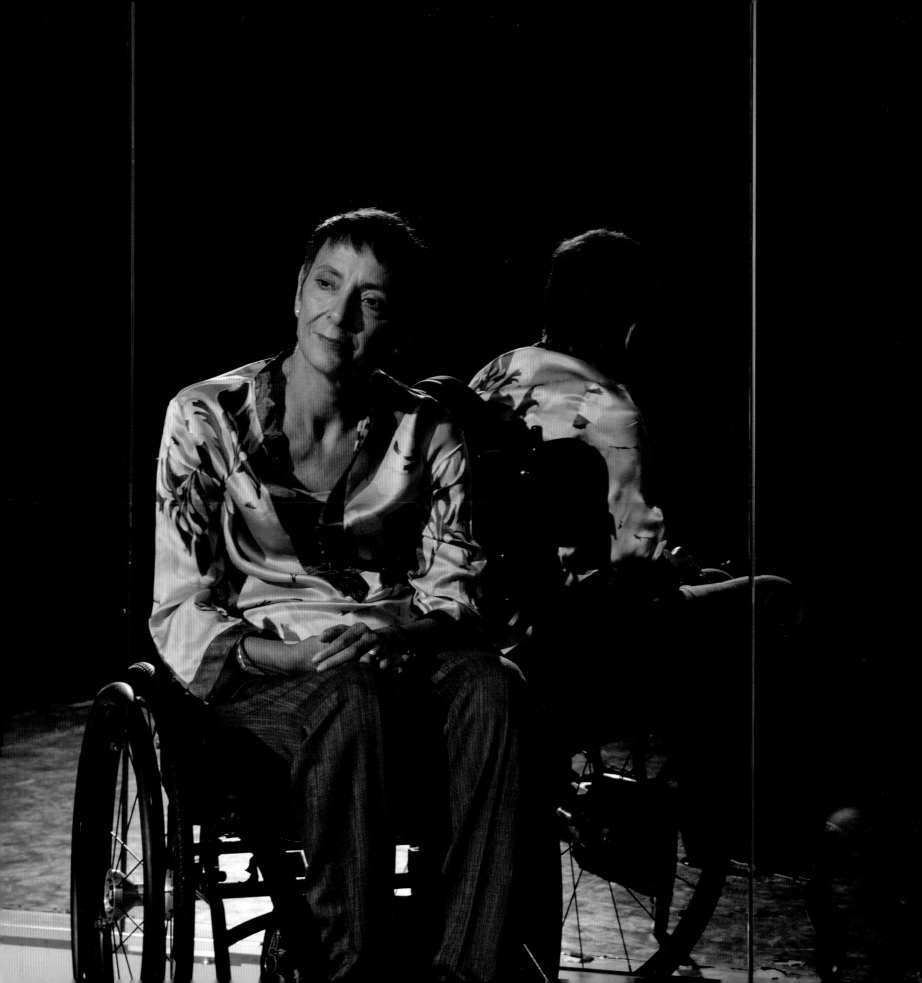

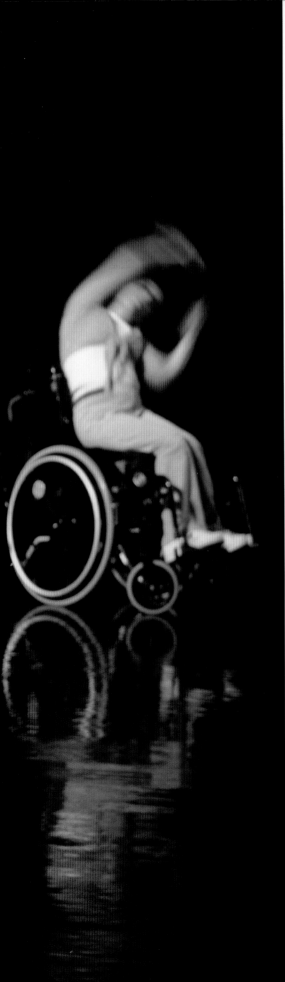

When I went to the Palace to collect my OBE for services to dance, the Queen asked, 'Do you do a lot of this sort of dancing?' She must have found the idea of a wheelchair user dancing hard to grasp. But then lots of people do.

I had set up CandoCo in 1991, with Adam Benjamin, as an integrated dance company for both disabled and non-disabled artists. It was in the gym at the Aspire National Training Centre that we began to explore how we could dance together with our different physicalities. Far from being limited, we were creative and pushed the boundaries of more formal and conventional dance techniques.

I'm very proud of what the company has achieved, and continues to achieve, teaching and performing all around the world, including at the closing ceremony for the 2008 Olympics and Paralympics in Beijing. In 2007 I retired as the Artistic Director but, as Founder and Patron, I continue to promote and support them.

Now I'm enjoying spending more time with my family and my husband, Trevor, who I married nine years ago.

We began to explore how we could dance together

He had been a boyfriend back in the late 1960s before I had my accident on stage in 1973 while performing with the London Contemporary Dance Company. We'd lost touch but he read an article about CandoCo and tracked me down. I'm also planning to take up some old hobbies again. Life drawing is now my passion and I can devote some time to a class. And we both love living in London and go out a lot, as well as doing a lot of cooking and entertaining together.

Over the years I have met some extraordinary people, through CandoCo and in everyday life. Many of my PAs have become good friends over the years and we still keep in contact. They have made my life easier, and some have been great fun to be with. I feel, with their assistance, that I have managed to continue leading as full and interesting a life as possible.

Like anyone else, I have my disappointments – apart from the obvious one. I would have liked children, but either the timing or relationship wasn't right. But I am now 'Granny Celeste' to Trevor's granddaughter, Sadie, who is wonderful and a great source of pleasure to us.

I remember one night, while I was still on the spinal unit, going to dinner at Buckingham Palace with my husband, Norman, who was in the Cabinet at the time. I was sitting opposite some rather stuffy European dignitaries and had a salad put in front of me. Salad is still one of the most difficult things for me to eat and I must have looked worried.

We ate our lettuce with our fingers

Then such a kind chap on my right, who I later discovered was the Master of the Queen's Household, spotted my embarrassment. He nudged me and said, "Come on, let's just do it!" Together we ate our lettuce with our fingers. The dignified ladies sitting opposite looked shocked, but I honestly don't think that the Queen would have minded. The boys on the ward roared with laughter when I came back that night and told them.

There was such camaraderie on the ward. I was about 50 years old then and there were lots of young boys there with me who were huge fun and very kind. I remember one trying to teach me chess. My son told him, "Don't bother, I've been trying to teach her for years."

The doctors wouldn't let me refer to the IRA bomb at the Grand Hotel in Brighton in 1984 that left me paralysed from just below my shoulders as an accident. They told me I had to call it a terrorist bomb which, of course, it was.

In hospital, and when I first came home, friends and family kept me going. It is a problem that I can't move my hands much and reading isn't easy as I can't turn the pages, but I love 'my' Classic FM and we sometimes go to the opera and live theatre. Perhaps one day they will make an electric book reader I can manage.

This year, I hope to have a new canine partner; he's a labradoodle and, since I'm unable to open doors, he will be trained to do that and very much more. Certainly, on the rare occasions that I am left on my own in the house, he will help me get about, but I will still need my two carers too. I love the garden and whether I'm outside or, if wet, inside looking out, I like to take an interest and see what's happening.

I have been fortunate enough throughout my life to meet some wonderful people. On one occasion, Nelson Mandela waved everyone away and said, "This is the girl I've come to meet."

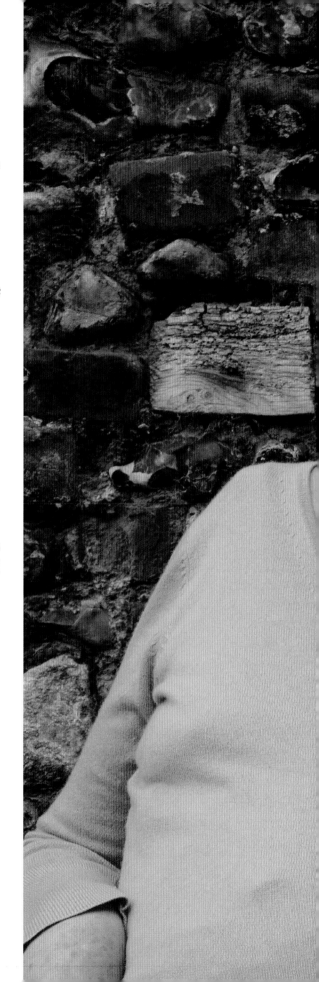

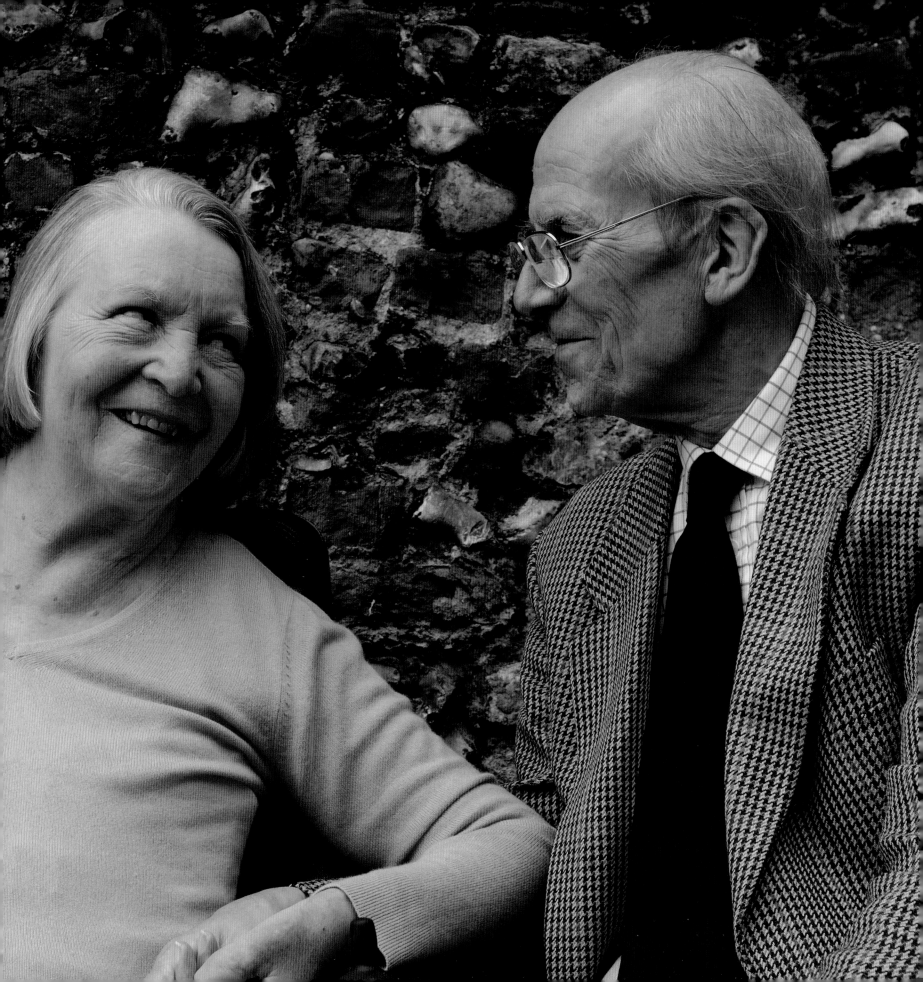

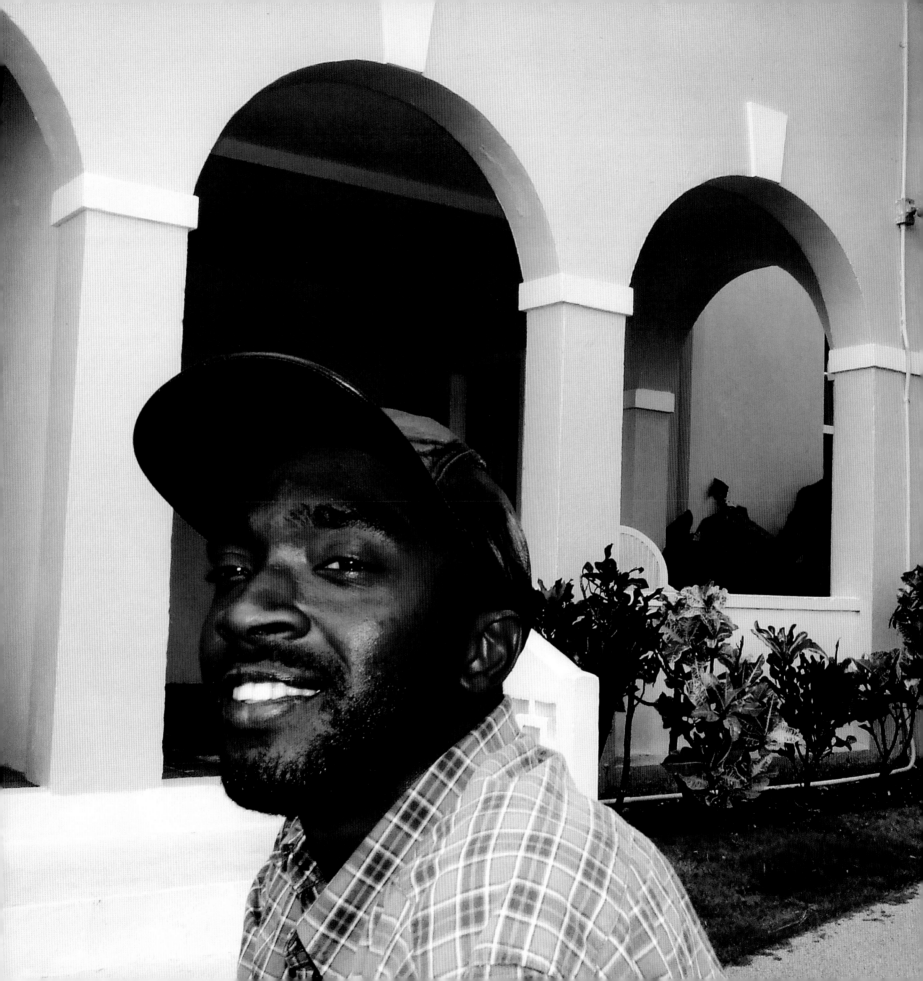

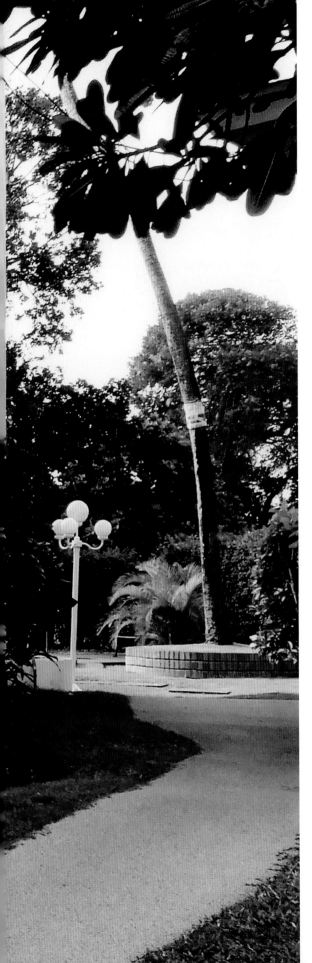

I spent 12 months in hospital here in Barbados after my accident. I was 11 and had been travelling with my family on the back seat of a car when there was a crash. The doctor waited until I was being discharged to tell me I would never walk again and never live a 'normal person's life'. I remember thinking, "This guy is crazy, I've known that for a year." After a few months in hospital, I'd already envisaged how my life would be and decided to get myself back to school, and begin to make and achieve my own goals.

The hospitals in Barbados do not provide rehabilitation or equipment unless you pay for it. My dad had to buy me my first wheelchair; it was the sort an old lady would sit in and so it did nothing for my image. Finally, a friend in Canada got me a Wheelie chair, which made all the difference to getting about. My school was not adapted but my friends were - they would carry me whenever I couldn't get somewhere. I know I have to depend on others, but when I hear people telling me I can't do something, I usually go away and work out a way that I can. I travelled with a friend to Mexico to participate in wheelchair sports and when we got back we set up the Paralympics Association of Barbados.

It's frustrating not to be able to drive myself about. I am always dependent on friends driving me, or the expense of taking taxis. My wish is that I am allowed to take my test, buy a car and be independent. It would also help me develop and expand my business as a designer and artist; I sell a lot of my work to the tourists who come out to the island and to the hotels as well.

My school was not adapted but my friends were

I enjoy female company a lot and have some very special ladies in my life who don't seem to mind about my being in a wheelchair at all. I believe in a degree of spirituality and that there is something greater in life. That helps me push on when things are tough.

I go in to the hospital here and talk to some of the patients and tell them life is not going to be as it was, but that they will be able to do things in some capacity. The fact is, no one can help you build willpower, you've got to do that yourself, but don't let disability be a limitation.

I was an apprentice electrician when I had my accident diving into a pool in Brazil. Afterwards, I thought I would do something different, as I had the time to study. My PA suggested I get myself to college and do accountancy. I wasn't even very good at maths but I gave it a shot. That was three years ago and now I'm an Associated Account Technician and also studying to become a chartered accountant.

Boys need their wheels

It was my family who helped me after my accident and stopped me getting depressed or unhappy. My brother's a DJ so I sometimes go clubbing, and I like socialising and having a good time with friends. Some of them have places of their own now so I go round to visit them or they come to me. I'm quite energetic and enjoy going to the gym, but if it's raining I don't usually go out. Wheelchairs and rain don't mix, and I don't drive – yet. But I will pass my driving test; boys need their wheels!

When I was away skiing a few years ago I broke my leg in a collision with a tree. It took a really long while to heal, almost a year, and it's not easy to get about with a great metal frame sticking straight out in front of you. I had to fight to keep the leg, but after lots of physio and finally corrective surgery, it's still there and I can now move it about more easily. Not sure I'll be going skiing again though, but if I do I'll be looking out for those trees.

My latest road trip was to the Czech Republic to visit some friends, and then on to Poland. We did all the touristy stuff, including going down a salt mine in Wielczcha. It meant dropping 100 metres underground by lift and then taking a further 500 steps (I bounced down in my chair) to the very bottom where there was a huge church carved out of the rock - quite amazing. I came back up in the lift from what felt like the centre of the earth.

Does volunteering count as a hobby? Because that's what I do up at Aspire, helping patients learn to use the computers in the IT suite and on the ward. I really enjoy helping them with their problems and coming up with ways to get them using the computers again, particularly when they've initially thought it's beyond their capabilities. I suppose when they meet me and see that I have a high level spinal injury they are reassured, because quite honestly it's true: if I can do it, so can they.

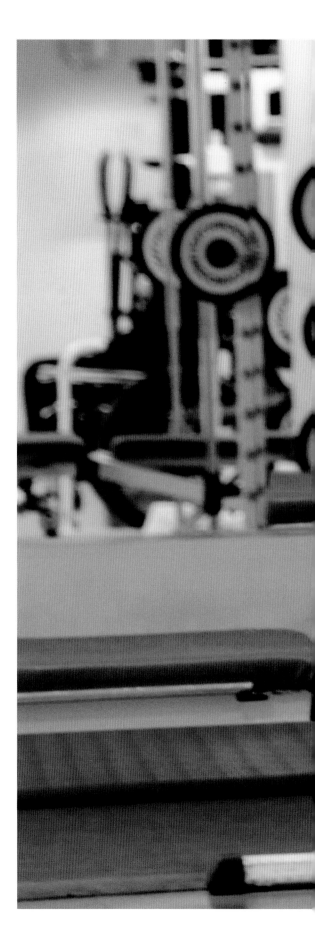

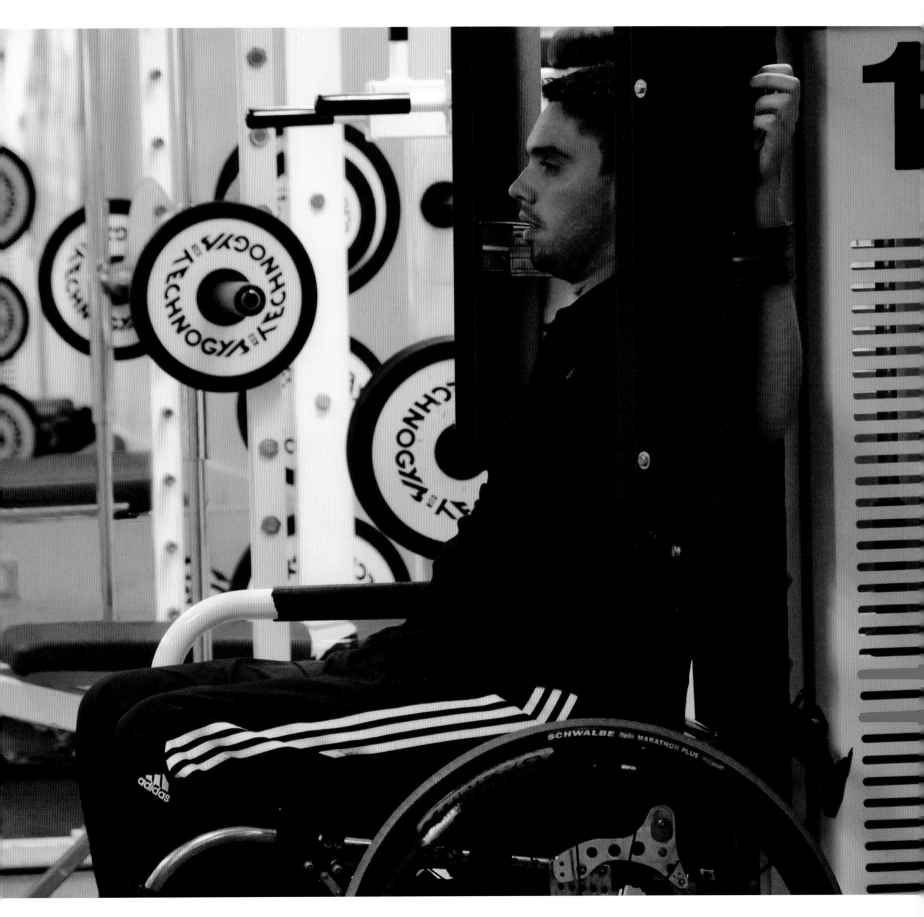

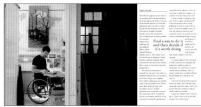

Tim Rushby-Smith Pages 4/5

Injured at 36

Fall

Rehab: Stoke Mandeville for 3 months

Injury Level: T12

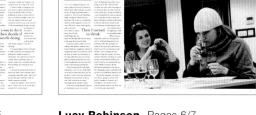

Lucy Robinson Pages 6/7

Injured at 18

Sailing accident overseas

Rehab: Stoke Mandeville for 9 months

Injury Level: C5/6

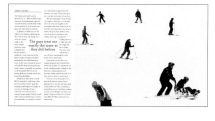

Andy Walker Pages 8/9

Injured at 28

Swimming accident overseas

Rehab: Delhi for 2 months,

Sheffield for 7 months

Injury Level: C4/5

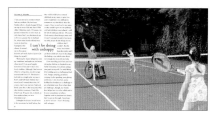

Lynne Daly Pages 10/11

Injured at 20

Fallen on

Rehab: Stanmore for 5 months

Injury Level: T12 complete/ L1 incomplete

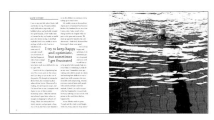

Jane Morley Pages 12/13

Paralysed at 65

Non-medical Trauma

Rehab: Devonshire Hospital,

London for 3 months

Injury Level: T11/12

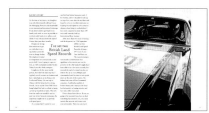

David Edwards Pages 16/17

Injured at 35

Road Traffic Accident (car)

Rehab: Stanmore for 3 months

Injury Level: C6/7

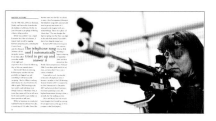

Mandy Pankhurst Pages 18/19

Injured at 42

Horse riding accident

Rehab: Stanmore for 8 months

Injury Level: T12 incomplete

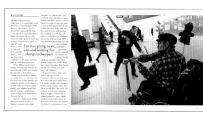

Max Reid Pages 20/21

Paralysed at 56

Non-Medical Trauma

Operated at The National Hospital for

Neurology & Neurosurgery, London

Injury Level: T12

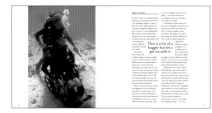

Michael Mackenzie Pages 22/23

Injured at 45

Road Traffic Accident (pedestrian)

Rehab: Stoke Mandeville for 14 months

Injury Level: T3

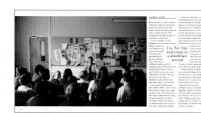

Andrew Stitson Pages 24/25

Injured at 29

Road Traffic Accident (pedestrian)

Rehab: Stanmore for 9 months

Injury Level: C5 incomplete

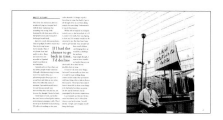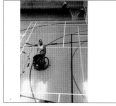

Brett Wainwright Pages 26/27

Injured at 26

Road Traffic Accident (motorbike)

Rehab: Stanmore for 3 months

Injury Level: T8

Joe Gilbert Pages 30/31

Injured at 19

Fall

Rehab: Oswestry for 6 months

Injury Level: T12/L1 incomplete

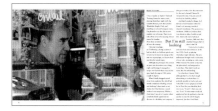

Rudi Breakwell-Bos Pages 32/33

Injured at 17

Skiing accident overseas

Rehab: Geneva for 4 months

Injury Level: C5/6

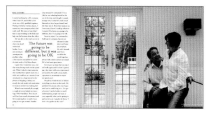

Reg Coote Pages 34/35

Injured at 39

Industrial injury

Rehab: Stanmore for 4 months

Injury Level: T1

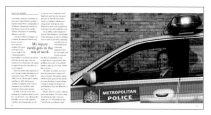

Paula Craig OBE Pages 36/37

Injured at 37

Road Traffic Accident (cycling)

Rehab: Stanmore for 5 months

Injury Level: T12

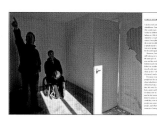

Luke Hamill Pages 38/39

Injured at 18

Road Traffic Accident (car)

Rehab: Stanmore for 5 months

Injury Level: T8

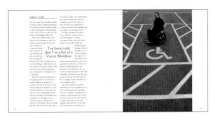

Barry Reed Pages 42/43

Injured at 32

Road Traffic Accident (motorbike)

Rehab: Stanmore for 6 months

Injury Level: T5

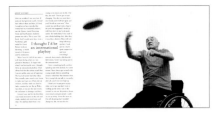

John Harris Pages 44/45

Injured at 19

Fall

Rehab: Stoke Mandeville for 5 months

Injury Level: L1

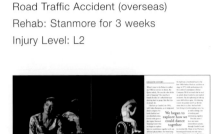

Sheike Sheike Pages 46/47

Injured at 6

Road Traffic Accident (overseas)

Rehab: Stanmore for 3 weeks

Injury Level: L2

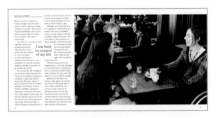

Mandi Peers Pages 48/49

Injured at 38

Road Traffic Accident (motorbike)

Rehab: Stanmore for 8 months

Injury Level: T4

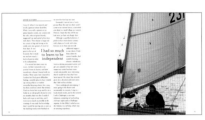

Anne Luttman-Johnson Pages 50/51

Injured at 21

Road Traffic Accident (Car)

Rehab: Salisbury for 6 months

Injury Level: T11

Celeste Dandeker MBE Pages 54/55

Injured at 22

Fall while dancing

Rehab: Ostwestry for 7 months

Injury Level: C5/6 incomplete

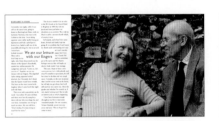

Lady Margaret Tebbit Pages 56/57

Injured at 50

Brighton Bombing

Rehab: Stoke Mandeville and Stanmore

for 2 years

Injury Level: C4

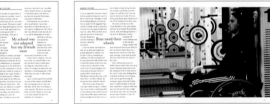
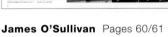

Junior Howe Pages 58/59

Injured at 11

Road Traffic Accident (car)

Rehab: Barbados for 12 months

Injury Level: L2

James O'Sullivan Pages 60/61

Injured at 17

Diving accident overseas

Rehab: Stanmore for 7 months

Injury Level: C5/6

Thank you

Aspire would like to thank everyone who has contributed, in whatever way, to making *It's My Life* possible.

We would especially like to thank those who took the time to tell us their stories and are featured in this book, but equally those with moving and encouraging words to say that, sadly, we were unable to use. This is their book, too.

Photography

All photographhy

Max Forsythe

www.maxforsythe.com

+44 (0)20 8948 6888

max@maxforsythe.com

Except pages 22,40/41 & 58/59

Design & Production

Frank Sully & Partners

+44 (0)20 7267 9747

frank-sully@btconnect.com

An Aspire publication

ISBN

978-0-9563371-0-8

It's my life

Printing

Oriental Press

All proceeds from this book will go to Aspire.

Registered

Charity No. 1075317

Scottish Registered

Charity No. SC037482

www.aspire.org.uk

Aspire is grateful to Hollister for their kind sponsorship of *It's My Life*.

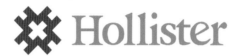

Hollister Limited is dedicated to delivering the highest standard of products and services in Ostomy Care and Continence Care. Each of our product lines is backed by a policy of unconditional customer satisfaction.

At Hollister, our Continence Care products are designed for people who have spinal cord injuries. Our continence product portfolio includes intermittent catheters, leg/night bags and more recently the Zassi Bowel Management System. As we continue to develop quality products and services, our goal remains the same, to promote control, independence and quality of life.